Advance Praise for *50 Studies Every Anesthesiologist Should Know*

"The authors provide a riveting summary of the 50 most influential and important papers in the field of anesthesiology. They dissect each study, discussing the strengths, weaknesses, and relevance of each. Some of the particularly compelling sections include pain medicine, critical care, regional anesthesia, and obstetrics. For anesthesiologists interested in an easy way to brush up on the literature and improve the care of their patients, this book will be a valuable addition to their collection."

—**Steven P. Cohen, MD**, Chief of Pain Medicine & Director of Clinical Operations,
Professor of Anesthesiology & Critical Care Medicine, Neurology and
Physical Medicine & Rehabilitation,
Johns Hopkins School of Medicine,
Director of Pain Research,
Walter Reed National Military Medical Center,
Professor of Anesthesiology and Physical Medicine & Rehabilitation,
Uniformed Services University of the Health Sciences,
Baltimore, MD

"The pace of medical innovation continues to accelerate and the growth in the published medical literature has reached the point that it is nearly impossible to keep up. As we strive to understand the relevance of new research evidence to guide our clinical practice, it is important to understand the foundation on which current recommendations are built and new studies are developed. *50 Studies Every Anesthesiologist Should Know* is a wonderful summary of articles relevant to clinical practice across the spectrum of anesthesiology practice. I highly recommend this to all current and future anesthesiologists."

—**Richard W. Rosenquist, MD**, Chairman, Department of Pain Management, Cleveland
Clinic, Cleveland, OH

"Dr. Anita Gupta is a visionary – a humanistic physician who is truly driven by the betterment of patients and society. She has a long-standing commitment to medical education and patient care, which helped shape this wonderfully useful book. I know it will serve to educate many students and physicians and help them to improve the lives of many patients for many years to come."

—**Stewart D. Friedman, PhD**, Practice Professor Emeritus,
The Wharton School, University of Pennsylvania, Philadelphia, PA

50 STUDIES EVERY DOCTOR SHOULD KNOW

50 Studies Every Doctor Should Know: The Key Studies that Form the Foundation of Evidence Based Medicine, Revised Edition
Michael E. Hochman

50 Studies Every Internist Should Know
Kristopher Swiger, Joshua R. Thomas, Michael E. Hochman, and Steven Hochman

50 Studies Every Neurologist Should Know
David Y. Hwang and David M. Greer

50 Studies Every Pediatrician Should Know
Ashaunta T. Anderson, Nina L. Shapiro, Stephen C. Aronoff, Jeremiah Davis, and Michael Levy

50 Imaging Studies Every Doctor Should Know
Christoph I. Lee

50 Studies Every Surgeon Should Know
SreyRam Kuy, Rachel J. Kwon, and Miguel A. Burch

50 Studies Every Intensivist Should Know
Edward A. Bittner

50 Studies Every Palliative Care Doctor Should Know
David Hui, Akhila Reddy, and Eduardo Bruera

50 Studies Every Psychiatrist Should Know
Ish P. Bhalla, Rajesh R. Tampi, and Vinod H. Srihari

50 Studies Every Anesthesiologist Should Know

EDITED BY

ANITA GUPTA, DO, PHARMD, MPP
Robertson Fellow and Liechtenstein Institute Fellow
Graduate Associate, Julius Rabinowitz Center for Public Policy and Finance
Woodrow Wilson School of Public and International Affairs
Princeton University
Princeton, NJ

CHAPTER EDITOR

ELENA N. GUTMAN, MD
Assistant Professor, Department of Anesthesiology
Yale School of Medicine
Yale University
New Haven, CT

SERIES EDITOR

MICHAEL E. HOCHMAN, MD, MPH
Associate Professor, Medicine
Director, Gehr Family Center for Health Systems Science
USC Keck School of Medicine
Los Angeles, CA

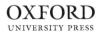

OXFORD
UNIVERSITY PRESS

OXFORD
UNIVERSITY PRESS

Oxford University Press is a department of the University of Oxford. It furthers
the University's objective of excellence in research, scholarship, and education
by publishing worldwide. Oxford is a registered trade mark of Oxford University
Press in the UK and certain other countries.

Published in the United States of America by Oxford University Press
198 Madison Avenue, New York, NY 10016, United States of America.

Library of Congress Cataloging-in-Publication Data
Names: Gupta, Anita, 1975– editor. | Gutman, Elena N., editor.
Title: 50 studies every anesthesiologist should know /
edited by Anita Gupta ; chapter editor, Elena N. Gutman.
Other titles: Fifty studies every anesthesiologist should know |
50 studies every doctor should know (Series)
Description: Oxford ; New York : Oxford University Press, [2019] |
Series: 50 studies every doctor should know | Includes bibliographical references and index.
Identifiers: LCCN 2018012948 | ISBN 9780190237691 (alk. paper)
Subjects: | MESH: Anesthesia—methods | Anesthesia—adverse effects |
Intraoperative Complications—prevention & control | Postoperative
Complications—prevention & control | Evidence-Based Medicine |
Clinical Trials as Topic
Classification: LCC RD81 | NLM WO 200 | DDC 617.9/6—dc23
LC record available at https://lccn.loc.gov/2018012948

9 8 7 6 5 4 3 2 1

Printed by Webcom, Inc., Canada

Dedicated to the beacons of my life, Sanjeev, Shaan, Jay, for their unconditional love.

—ANITA GUPTA

CONTENTS

SECTION 3 Neuroanesthesia

SECTION 4 Critical Care

SECTION 5 Perioperative Medicine

SECTION 6 Pain Anesthesiology

SECTION 7 Regional Anesthesiology

SECTION 8 Obstetric Anesthesiology

SECTION 9 Pediatric Anesthesiology

FOREWORD FROM THE SERIES EDITOR

When I was a third-year medical student, I asked one of my senior residents—who seemed to be able to quote every medical study in the history of mankind—if he had a list of key studies that have defined the current practice of general medicine which I should read before graduating medical school. "Don't worry," he told me. "You will learn the key studies as you go along."

But picking up on these key studies didn't prove so easy and I was frequently admonished by my attendings for being unaware of crucial literature in their field. More importantly, because I had a mediocre understanding of the medical literature at that time, I lacked confidence in my clinical decision-making and had difficulty appreciating the significance of new research findings. It wasn't until I was well into my residency— thanks to considerable amount of effort and determination—that I finally began to feel comfortable with both the emerging and fundamental medical literature.

Now, as a practicing general internist, I realize that I am not the only doctor who has struggled to become familiar with the key medical studies that form the foundation of evidence-based practice. Many of the students and residents I work with tell me that they feel overwhelmed by the medical literature, and that they cannot process new research findings because they lack a solid understanding of what has already been published. Even many practicing physicians—including those with years of experience—have only a cursory knowledge of the medical evidence base and make clinical decisions largely on personal experience.

I initially wrote *50 Studies Every Doctor Should Know* in an attempt to provide medical professionals (and even lay readers interested in learning more about medical research) a quick way to get up to speed on the classic studies that shape clinical practice. But it soon became clear there was a greater need for this distillation of the medical evidence than my original book provided. Soon after the book's publication, I began receiving calls from specialist physicians in a variety of disciplines wondering about the possibility of another book focusing on studies in their field. In partnership with a wonderful team of editors from Oxford University Press, we have developed my initial book into a series, offering volumes in Internal Medicine, Pediatrics, Surgery, Neurology, Radiology, Critical Care Medicine, and now Anesthesia. Several additional volumes are in the works.

I am particularly excited about this latest volume in Anesthesia, which is the culmination of hard work by two dedicated editors – Anita Gupta and Elena Gutman, who worked tirelessly to identify and summarize the most important studies in their field. There tend to be fewer rigorous randomized trials in the field of Anesthesia than in some other medical disciplines. Nevertheless, Drs. Gupta and Gutman found studies that offer important lessons on the central topics in their field. I believe *50 Studies Every Anesthesiologist Should Know* provides the perfect launching ground for trainees in the field as well as a helpful refresher for practicing clinicians – physicians, nurse anesthetists, and other anesthesia professionals. The book also highlights key knowledge gaps that may stimulate researchers to tackle key unanswered questions in the field. A special thanks also goes to the wonderful editors at Oxford University Press – Andrea Knobloch and Emily Samulski – who injected energy and creativity into the production process for this volume. This volume was a pleasure to help develop, and I learned a lot about the field of Anesthesia in the process.

I have no doubt you will gain important insights into the field of Anesthesiology in the pages ahead!

Michael E. Hochman, MD, MPH

FOREWORD

Over the past several decades, there has been a movement from eminence-based care to evidence-based care. This has occurred in numerous specialties although the number and size of the clinical trials upon which to base care has varied greatly between specialties such as cardiology where mega trials have become common to anesthesiology where until recently much of the evidence base is smaller trials or closed claims given the incidence of rare outcomes such as anesthetic – related mortality. Importantly, the evidence base for anesthesiology has grown dramatically and there are numerous critical papers which help shape today's best practices. Dr. Anita Gupta has added to the series of books published by Oxford on the 50 Studies Every Doctor Should Know by the inclusion of anesthesiology. She has used a templated approach in which her contributors have assessed the quality of the study, limitations and implications. This will allow the readers to better understand the database and make their own decisions on how it should be incorporated into care. Dr. Anita Gupta is the ideal individual to edit this book with her expertise in pain management, pharmacology and additional training through her Masters in Public Policy. Her recent experience that Princeton University's Woodrow Wilson School of Public Health and International Affairs and work with the World Health Organization further provides are with the expertise to put together this important publication. This book should help all anesthesiologists improve their understanding of the literature and therefore the practice of evidence-based medicine.

Lee A. Fleisher, MD
Robert D. Dripps Professor and Chair of Anesthesiology and Critical Care
Perelman School of Medicine of the University of Pennsylvania
Philadelphia, PA

FOREWORD

I met Dr. Anita Gupta for the first time when she had just begun her health policy studies at the Woodrow Wilson School of Public Policy and International Affairs at Princeton University. She had decided to pause in the midst of a thriving career as an anesthesiologist at a major academic medical school in order to study health policy related to the ongoing opioid epidemic in Philadelphia. As I recall, I could not suppress my surprise that an anesthesiologist would make such a bold and progressive career move. She looked past my obvious bias, and explained that it was <u>because</u> of her career as an anesthesiologist that she felt a special purpose. Her goal was to leverage her professional experience with training at a premier university towards changing public policy in a way that is evidence-informed. She was persuasive in her conviction that physicians who understood the evidence base and had been on the front line of combating the epidemic were in dire need as policy makers. She made perfect sense, and I learned not to question one's motives based on professional discipline. It was equally impressive that she had chosen perhaps the most rigorous program in the country to learn public policy. This too eventually made perfect sense, for as I came to know all too well, Dr. Gupta is not one to make a major decision without learning all that she could from the available evidence.

The evidence base is our guide, but there cannot possibly be a randomized control trial for each and every decision. When I learned that Dr. Gupta and her co-editors had spent years compiling a tome of fifty of the most critical studies for anesthesiologists, my first thought was that, yet again, this made perfect sense. This book serves as a guide for clinicians who must translate the best available evidence to unique clinical scenarios. Understanding why a study is important is sometimes the easy part- the art of medicine involves translating that study to inform real-life decisions that we, and more importantly, our patients, face every day. My supposition is that there is special value in learning from the perspective of a gifted and skilled physician. My hope is that the reader keep in mind that the Dr. Gupta's voice is informed by her professional <u>as well as</u> her life experience. She teaches us that we, as physicians, have a special responsibility to be as skilled in translating the available evidence as we hope all doctors will be.

Jonathan R. Pletcher, MD
Director, Medical Services
University Health Services
Princeton University
Princeton, NJ

PREFACE

Do you remember the first day of medical school? It may be hard for many to recall all the details of the day, but when you ask physicians, most will remember how they felt. Usually, they will say that they recalled being excited, ambitious, and slightly nervous but overwhelmingly optimistic and filled with compassion for the patients we were about to take on. When I set out to compile this book, I thought about how pivotal it is to understand that what we feel on the first day of medical school should be how we feel every day and lifelong as a physician even with the rapidly changing world of medicine. To further this, physicians need to have a strong foundation of evidence so that we can always offer our patients the best possible care with the most amount of empathy, which often leads to better patient outcomes. Understanding evidence in medicine can be time-consuming and often cumbersome given the growing demands of the field, and much of those feelings of excitement may become fleeting very quickly with the inundation of required tasks.

To understand the evidence, physicians must have access to clear, concise, organized, and clinically relevant information. This book provides exactly that. I attempted to curate and organize information that can be critically important for any anesthesiologist anywhere in the world. This book summarizes the most relevant information in a concisely in a few pages for some of the most current and influential studies in our specialty.

How were the studies selected? It was by no means easy. Hundreds of landmark studies were narrowed down to the final 50. Numerous anesthesiologists reviewed the selections to determine the studies that should be included. There is no perfect way to decide which studies are the most critical. By the end of the selection process, it came down to what matters most to anesthesiologists and what may have a significant impact on our patients. In most cases, it came down to knowing which evidence may affect a patient's life for all anesthesiologists. The most relevant studies were the final 50 that are included here for you to review.

I genuinely hope that you will find this book as informative as I have when preparing it over years of careful and diligent curation. I believe this book will help your practice and your understanding of how valuable evidence is essential to our work every day and to the care of our patients' lives and their families. This evidence can help us to be compassionate, ambitious, and optimistic about every patient we treat and to ensure we are delivering the best medical care with the utmost empathy and evidence in hand as we take on the practice of medicine each and every day as anesthesiologists.

ACKNOWLEDGMENTS

I would like to acknowledge the countless individuals who have assisted with this book and many that have provided their insight and support to make this book a success.

I would like to thank Oxford University Press Senior Editor Andrea Knobloch, Associate Editor Rebecca Suzan, and Associate Editor Emily Samulski for making this book come to fruition and for their consistent vision and limitless encouragement, advice, and support. Andrea Knobloch is a true visionary, and I am proud to be an author with her mentorship. She has undoubtedly provided guidance to me both as a senior editor and mentor and as a friend through the many turns of life, and I am grateful that she has stood by every turn of this book to achieve its ultimate successful publication.

I would also like to thank my countless mentors over the years from all the institutions in which I have had the honor to learn anesthesiology, pain medicine, and health policy—Princeton University, Johns Hopkins University, Georgetown University, and the National Institutes of Health. Thank you for supporting my passion to advocate for change and to have an impact on public health, providing the best possible care to patients. And, thank you for truly making me understand the critical importance of strong evidence-based medicine, innovation, and policy to ensure that the change we make is always in the best interest of our patients.

I would like to thank the many esteemed faculty, graduate students, and medical students at the University of Pennsylvania School of Medicine, Drexel University College of Medicine, the University of Medicine and Dentistry of New Jersey, and most important, the American Society of Anesthesiologists for their endless support. This book would not be possible without their guidance and their ability to foster within me key leadership skills and a clear understanding of the importance of high-level evidence for delivering the highest level of medical care possible to patients.

I want to sincerely thank all the first authors of the 50 selected studies included in this book who generously reviewed the summaries for accuracy and complete-ness. I very much appreciate the assistance of these esteemed individuals. More important, I want to thank them for their dedication, commitment, and fine con-tribution to advancing the science of medicine, anesthesiology, critical care, and pain medicine.

1. The GlideScope Video Laryngoscope: randomized clinical trial in 200 patients. First author, D. A. Sun.
2. Management of the difficult airway: a closed claims analysis. First author, G. N. Peterson.
3. Incidence and predictors of difficult and impossible mask ventilation. First author, S. Kheterpal.
4. Perioperative maintenance of normothermia reduces the incidence of morbid cardiac events. A randomized clinical trial. First author, S. M. Frank.
5. Perioperative normothermia to reduce the incidence of surgical-wound infection and shorten hospitalization. First author, A. Kurz.
6. Preventable anesthesia mishaps: a study of human factors. First author, J. B. Cooper.
7. A randomized clinical trial of the effect of deliberate perioperative increase of oxygen delivery on mortality in high-risk surgical patients. First author, O. Boyd.
8. Effects of intensive glucose lowering in type 2 diabetes. First author, H. C. Gerstein.
9. Evaluation study of congestive heart failure and pulmonary artery catheterization effectiveness: the ESCAPE trial. First author, C. Binanay.
10. A comparison of rate control and rhythm control in patients with atrial fibrillation. First author, D. G. Wyse.
11. Early use of the pulmonary artery catheter and outcomes in patients with shock and acute respiratory distress syndrome. First author, C. Richard.
12. Statins decrease perioperative cardiac complications in patients undergoing noncardiac vascular surgery: the Statins for Risk Reduction in Surgery (StaRRS) study. First author, K. O'Neil-Callahan.
13. Safety of transesophageal echocardiography: a multicenter survey of 10,419 examinations. First author, W. G. Daniel.
14. Coronary revascularization in context. First author, R. A. Lange.

15. Effects of extended-release metoprolol succinate in patients undergoing non-cardiac surgery (POISE trial): a randomised controlled trial. First author, P. J. Devereaux.

16. Adverse cerebral outcomes after coronary bypass surgery. First author, G. W. Roach.

17. Long-term cognitive impairment after critical illness. First author, P. P. Pandharipande.

18. Cerebral perfusion pressure: management protocol and clinical results. First author, M. Rosner.

19. An intervention to decrease catheter-related bloodstream infections in the ICU. First author, P. Pronovost.

20. Early goal-directed therapy in the treatment of severe sepsis and septic shock. First author, E. Rivers.

21. Intensive insulin therapy and pentastarch resuscitation in severe sepsis. First author, F. Brunkhorst.

22. A multicenter, randomized, controlled clinical trial of transfusion requirements in critical care. First author, P. C. Hébert.

23. Effects of intravenous fluid restriction on postoperative complications: comparison of two perioperative fluid regimens: a randomized assessor-blinded multicenter trial. First author, B. Brandstrup.

24. A comparison of albumin and saline for fluid resuscitation in the intensive care unit. First author, S. Finfer.

25. Prevention of intraoperative awareness in a high-risk surgical population. First author, M. S. Avidan.

26. Evaluation of perioperative medication errors and adverse drug events. First author, K. C. Nanji.

27. A surgical safety checklist to reduce morbidity and mortality in a global population. First author, A. B. Haynes.

28. A factorial trial of six interventions for the prevention of postoperative nausea and vomiting. First author, C. C. Apfel.

29. Pronounced, episodic oxygen desaturation in the postoperative period: its association with ventilatory pattern and analgesic regimen. First author, D. M. Catley.

30. Surgical site infections following ambulatory surgery procedures. First author, P. L. Owens.

31. A reengineered hospital discharge program to decrease rehospitalization. First author, B. W. Jack.

32. Clinical significance of pulmonary aspiration during the perioperative period. First author, M. A. Warner.

33. Postoperative pain experience: results from a national survey suggest postoperative pain continues to be undermanaged. First author, J. L. Apfelbaum.
34. An fMRI-based neurologic signature of physical pain. First author, T. D. Wager.
35. Clinical importance of changes in chronic pain intensity measured on an 11-point numerical pain rating scale. First author, J. T. Farrar.
36. The induction and maintenance of central sensitization is dependent on N-methyl-D-aspartic acid receptor activation: implications for the treatment of post-injury pain hypersensitivity states. First author, C. J. Woolf.
37. Randomised trial of oral morphine for chronic non-cancer pain. First author, D. E. Moulin.
38. A randomized trial of epidural glucocorticoid injections for spinal stenosis. First author, J. L. Friedly.
39. Rapid magnetic resonance imaging vs radiographs for patients with low back pain: a randomized controlled trial. First author, J. G. Jarvik.
40. Randomised controlled trial to compare surgical stabilization of the lumbar spine with an intensive rehabilitation programme for patients with chronic lower back pain: the MRC spine stabilisation trial. First author, J. Fairbank.
41. Preoperative multimodal analgesia facilitates recovery after ambulatory laparoscopic cholecystectomy. First author, C. Mikaloliakou.
42. Reduction of postoperative mortality and morbidity with epidural or spinal anaesthesia: results from overview of randomised trials. First author, A. Rodgers.
43. Epidural anaesthesia and analgesia and outcome of major surgery: a randomised trial. First author, J. R. Rigg.
44. Nerve stimulator and multiple injection technique for upper and lower limb blockade: failure rate, patient acceptance, and neurologic complications. First author, G. Fanelli.
45. The risk of cesarean delivery with neuraxial analgesia given early versus late in labor. First author, C. A. Wong.
46. PDPH is a common complication of neuraxial blockade in parturients: a meta-analysis of obstetrical studies. First author, P. T. Choi.
47. Parental presence during induction of anesthesia versus sedative premedication: which intervention is more effective? First author, Z. N. Kain.

48. Pediatric anesthesia morbidity and mortality in the perioperative period. First author, M. M. Cohen.

49. CRIES: a new neonatal postoperative pain measurement score. Initial testing of validity and reliability. First author, S. W. Krechel.

50. Emergence agitation after sevoflurane versus propofol in pediatric patients. First author, S. Uezono.

SPECIAL THANKS

Hawa Abubaker, MD*
Washington University—St. Louis

Hemanth Adhar Baboolal, MD
University of North Carolina

Edward A. Bittner, MD, PhD,
FCCP, FCCM
Massachusetts General Hospital

Michelle Braunfeld, MD
University of California—Los Angeles

Jack C. Buckley, MD
University of California—Los Angeles

Steven P. Cohen, MD
Johns Hopkins University

Eleni H. Demas, BS*
United Nations, Paris, France

Brian Egan, MD, MPH
Columbia University

Nabil Elkassabany, MD
University of Pennsylvania

Michael A. Erdek, MD
Johns Hopkins University

Michael S. Green, DO
Drexel University College of Medicine

Melissa Haehn, MD
University of California—San
    Francisco

Michelle Harvey, MD
University of California—Los Angeles

Richard Hong, MD
University of California—Los Angeles

Mia Kang, MD
University of North Carolina

Nimit Lad, MD*
Temple University College of
    Medicine

Vipin Mehta, MD
Massachusetts General Hospital

Scott A. Miller, MD
Wake Forest University

Vicki Modest, MD
Massachusetts General Hospital

Robert Pluscec, MD*
Yale University

Sadeq A. Quraishi, MD, MHA, MMSc
Massachusetts General Hospital

Vendhan Ramanunjum, MD*
Drexel University College of Medicine

A. Sassan Sabouri, MD
Massachusetts General Hospital

Lu Zheng, MD*
University of Pittsburgh

Keren Ziv, MD
Drexel University College of Medicine

*Graduate researcher/assistant.

SECTION 1

General Anesthesiology

1

Video vs. Direct Laryngoscopy

A Randomized Clinical Trial

In most patients, the GlideScope® provided a laryngoscopic view equal to or better than that of direct laryngoscopy, but it took an additional 16 [seconds] (average) for tracheal intubation.

—Sun et al.[1]

Research Question: How does the GlideScope® Video Laryngoscope compare with direct laryngoscopy (DL) in terms of laryngoscopic view and time required for intubation?

Year Study Began: 2003.

Year Study Published: 2005.

Study Location: University of British Columbia in Vancouver, Canada.

Who Was Studied: Adult patients presenting for elective surgery during which tracheal intubation was indicated.

Who Was Excluded: Patients requiring rapid sequence induction or those with elevated intracranial pressure, known airway pathology, or cervical spine injury.

How Many Patients: 200.

Study Overview: See Figure 1.1 for an overview of the study's design.

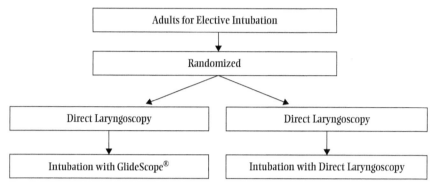

Figure 1.1 Summary of the study design.

Study Intervention: Following a standardized induction of general anesthesia and administration of nondepolarizing muscle relaxants, all patients underwent an initial DL with a Macintosh size 3 blade by a separate anesthetist not involved in subsequent intubations or patient care. For tracheal intubations, patients were intubated using either the GlideScope® or DL (randomization occurred before induction). The initial and intubation Cormack and Lehane[2] (C&L) laryngoscopy grades were recorded. Anesthetists responsible for intubations were blinded to the initial C&L grade. Total time to intubation (TTI) was noted. TTI was defined as the time the intubating instrument entered the patient's mouth until end-tidal carbon dioxide was detected. If more than one intubation attempt was required, the patient received bag-and-mask ventilation between attempts, and this time was not recorded as part of TTI.

Endpoints: Primary outcome: difference in C&L laryngoscopic score between DL and GlideScope®. Secondary outcomes: comparison of TTI between DL and GlideScope® with respect to C&L grades and airway measurements.

RESULTS

- Patient characteristics and airway parameters were similar in the two study groups.
- In the DL group, there was a high level of agreement between initial and intubating C&L laryngoscopy grades.
- There was a significant relationship between increasing Mallampati (MP) class[3] and decreasing thyromental distance (TMD) with the

initial C&L grades, but not with body mass index (BMI). There was no relationship between MP class, TMD, or BMI with TTI scores.

- There was an increase in TTI with increasing C&L grade in the DL group but not in the GlideScope® group. The overall mean TTI in the GlideScope® group was greater by 16 seconds compared with the DL group, reflecting a 50% increase; this difference was primarily due to C&L grade 1 and 2 patients. For C&L grade 3 patients, the difference in TTI between the two study groups was not significant.
- The majority of patients showed improvement in the C&L grade ($P <$ 0.001) obtained with the GlideScope® compared with DL. Notably, 14 of the 15 C&L grade 3 patients had an improved laryngoscopic grade with the GlideScope®.
- Nine patients required more than one attempt at intubation (three in the DL group and six in the GlideScope® group). For the six cases in the GlideScope® group requiring multiple intubation attempts, a good view of the larynx was seen on the monitor, but there was difficulty in directing the endotracheal tube (ETT) into the larynx.

Criticisms and Limitations: This study was terminated early at 200 patients when the data demonstrated a difference in the GlideScope® view (primary outcome measure). In order to achieve adequate power to demonstrate statistical equivalence between DL and GlideScope® intubations using TTI (accepted difference of ≤30 seconds) as an outcome measure, a further 250 patients would have been required.

Other Relevant Studies and Information:

- An observational study compared first-pass success rates using a Macintosh or Miller-style laryngoscope with the GlideScope®. Propensity scoring was used to select 626 subjects matched between the two groups based on multiple factors (e.g., MP class, cervical range of motion, mouth opening, dentition, weight, and past intubation history). For first-pass intubation attempts, DL was successful 80.8%, while the GlideScope® was successful 93.6% of the time ($P < 0.001$). After initial failure with DL, the GlideScope® was found to be 99% successful at intubation.[4]
- Given the occasional difficulty with directing the ETT into the larynx despite a good view during GlideScope® use, a recent randomized controlled trial of 160 patients requiring tracheal intubation for elective

surgery assessed whether orotracheal intubation with the GlideScope®
is faster and/or easier with inserting the ETT into the mouth before the
GlideScope®. No statistically significant difference was observed in the
time to intubate or the subjective ease of intubation whether the ETT or
GlideScope® was inserted into the oropharynx first.[5]

• The American Society of Anesthesiologists (ASA) Practice Guidelines
for Management of the Difficult Airway included information from
meta-analyses of randomized controlled trials comparing video-assisted
laryngoscopy with DL in patients with predicted or simulated difficult
airways. Video-assisted laryngoscopy yielded improved laryngeal
views and higher frequencies of successful intubations and first attempt
intubations. No differences in TTI, airway trauma, lip/gum trauma,
dental trauma, or sore throat were reported.[6]

Summary and Implications: This was the first randomized trial evaluating the
GlideScope® in comparison with the Macintosh laryngoscope. The GlideScope®
was designed to provide a view of the glottis without alignment of the oral, pharyngeal, and laryngeal axes. In most patients, the GlideScope® yielded improved
laryngoscopic views compared with DL, especially in the C&L grade 3 patients,
demonstrating an advantage over DL for difficult intubations. The increase in intubation time in C&L grade 1 and 2 patients and increased chance of multiple
intubation attempts suggest that the GlideScope® may not be the first-line choice
in patients with no contraindication to conventional laryngoscopy. The video laryngoscope has become an important modality for airway management.

CLINICAL CASE: VIDEO LARYNGOSCOPY

Case History

A 59-year-old man presents for elective laparoscopic hernia repair under general anesthesia with planned tracheal intubation. The patient has a history of
one prior surgical procedure. Review of the anesthetic record indicates the patient was a grade 1 mask ventilation but that two attempts were required for
intubation by two different providers using a Macintosh size 3 blade, and that
in both cases, the laryngoscopic view was C&L grade 3. Since the prior surgical procedure, the patient has gained 40 kg. Knowing this information, how
should the patient's airway be managed during intubation?

Suggested Answer

There are multiple options to prepare for endotracheal intubation in this patient. Given a history of difficult intubation with DL in the setting of additional weight gain, video laryngoscopy would likely offer improvement in the C&L view. Alternatively, a Bougie could be used. Laryngeal mask airways, a fiberoptic bronchoscope, and an additional anesthesia provider should be readily available if needed.

References

1. Sun DA, Warriner CB, Parsons DG, Klein R, Umedaly HS, Moult M. The GlideScope Video Laryngoscope: randomized clinical trial in 200 patients. *Br J Anaesth*. 2005 Mar;94(3):381–4.
2. Cormack RS, Lehane J. Difficult tracheal intubation in obstetrics. *Anaesthesia*. 1984 Nov;39(11):1105–11.
3. Mallampati SR, Gatt SP, Gugino LD, et al. A clinical sign to predict difficult tracheal intubation: a prospective study. *Can Anaesth Soc J*. 1985 Jul;32(4):429–34.
4. Ibinston JW, Ezaru CS, Cormican DS, Mangione MP. GlideScope use improves intubation success rates: an observational study using propensity score matching. *BMC Anesthesiol*. 2014 Nov 5;14:101.
5. Turkstra TP, Cusano F, Fridfinnson JA, Batohi P, Rachinsky M. Early endotracheal tube insertion with the GlideScope: a randomized controlled trial. *Anesth Analg*. 2016 Mar;122(3):753–7.
6. Apfelbaum JL, Hagberg CA, Caplan RA, et al. Practice guidelines for management of the difficult airway: an updated report by the American Society of Anesthesiologists Task Force on Management of the Difficult Airway. *Anesthesiology*. 2013 Feb;118(2):251–70.

2

Management of the Difficult Airway

A Closed Claims Analysis

Death [or brain damage] in claims from difficult airway management associated with induction of anesthesia but not other phases of anesthesia decreased in 1993–1999 compared with 1985–1992.

—Peterson et al.[1]

Research Question: What are the patterns of liability associated with malpractice claims arising from cases involving difficult airway management?

Funding: American Society of Anesthesiologists (ASA).

Year Study Began: 1985.

Year Study Published: 2005.

Study Location: The ASA Closed Claims Project (structured evaluation of adverse anesthetic outcomes obtained from the closed claims files of 35 professional liability insurance companies representing anesthesiologists from all over the United States).

Who Was Studied: ASA Closed Claims difficult airway management cases occurring between 1985 and 1999.

How Many Patients: 179 cases.

Study Overview: See Figure 2.1 for an overview of the study's design.

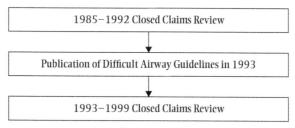

| 1985–1992 Closed Claims Review |
| Publication of Difficult Airway Guidelines in 1993 |
| 1993–1999 Closed Claims Review |

Figure 2.1 Summary of the study design.

Study Intervention: A retrospective review of difficult airway claims in the ASA Closed Claims database was conducted using a standardized data collection method. Two time periods (1985–1992 and 1993–1999) spanned before and after publication of the ASA Guidelines for the Management of the Difficult Airway in 1993.[2] Patient and case characteristics, outcomes, liability, and risk factors for death or brain damage (death/BD) were compared.

Endpoints: Airway management, outcomes, and the role of the 1993 Difficult Airway Guidelines in litigation.

RESULTS

- Of the 179 difficult airway claims, 48% ($n = 86$) were from events in 1985–1992 and 52% ($n = 93$) were from 1993–1999. Patient and case characteristics were similar in the two time periods except for the proportion of emergency surgery.
- The majority of claims ($n = 156$) involved perioperative care (on induction, during surgery, at extubation, or during recovery), and 13% ($n = 23$) involved outside locations (example: intensive care unit). Of the perioperative care claims, 67% occurred during induction, 15% during surgery, 12% at extubation, and 5% during recovery.
- Death/BD occurred in all outside location claims and more than half of perioperative claims. Difficult mask ventilation and the development of an airway emergency increased the odds of death/BD.
- In claims where an emergency airway situation developed, outcomes were worse with persistent attempts at intubation before attempting emergency nonsurgical ventilation or surgical airway access.

- Awake intubation was attempted but was unsuccessful in 12 claims, resulting in death/BD in 75%. Two clinical scenarios of awake intubation predisposed to poor outcomes: sedation/airway instrumentation in the presence of pharyngeal infection and induction of anesthesia after unsuccessful attempts at awake intubation due to technical problems or lack of patient cooperation.
- The majority of extubation or recovery claims were associated with a difficult intubation on induction, obesity, and/or sleep apnea.
- The proportion of claims where induction of anesthesia resulted in death/BD significantly decreased in 1993–1999 (35%) compared with 1985–1992 (62%).
- There was no difference in liability in the two time periods or between perioperative and outside location claims. Payment was made in more than half of the difficult airway claims. For 1993–1999, the Difficult Airway Guidelines were discussed in 18% of claims and were used to both defend and criticize care.

Criticisms and Limitations: This retrospective review lacks denominator data, making cause-and-effect relationships between events and changes in practice difficult to establish. The relative safety/efficacy of rescue techniques for management of the difficult airway cannot be estimated. There is case selection bias because of the presence of severe injury and substandard care leading to litigation. The time delay between injury occurrence and case appearance within the database (estimated at 3–6 years) makes evaluating the effect of training or new technology (e.g., fiberoptic bronchoscopy) on liability difficult.

Other Relevant Studies and Information:

- Studies have demonstrated repeated tracheal intubation attempts with direct laryngoscopy in emergency airway situations to be associated with airway and hemodynamic adverse events, suggesting that advanced airway devices or alternative airway rescue techniques should be considered after three unsuccessful direct laryngoscopy attempts.[3]
- The ASA Task Force on Management of the Difficult Airway published the most recent Practice Guidelines for Management of the Difficult Airway in February of 2013. The guidelines list recommendations for airway evaluation, preparation for difficult airway management,

strategies and recommendations for intubation and extubation, and recommendations for follow-up care.[4]

Summary and Implications: Although this is a retrospective review, analysis of difficult airway claims demonstrated a reduction in death or brain damage with induction of anesthesia in 1993–1999 compared with 1985–1992, suggesting that the Difficult Airway Guidelines published in 1993 improved airway management planning in cases with anticipated difficult airways. Since 1993, the ASA Difficult Airway Guidelines have been used to both defend and criticize care in litigation.

CLINICAL CASE: DIFFICULT AIRWAY MANAGEMENT

Case History

A 45-year-old man is undergoing a laparoscopic cholecystectomy. The patient is obese and has obstructive sleep apnea and a short, thick neck. You are taking over anesthetic care in the operating room shortly after incision. The anesthesia provider reports that the patient was a grade 3 mask ventilation and a difficult intubation. The vocal cords and arytenoid cartilages were unable to be visualized with direct laryngoscopy using Macintosh size 3 and 4 blades. A laryngeal mask airway was then placed, and the patient was ventilated until a video laryngoscope was obtained. Using a video laryngoscope size 3 blade yielded a grade 3 view, but the endotracheal tube was unable to be passed through the vocal cords. A subsequent attempt using a video laryngoscope size 4 blade and repositioning the patient's head yielded a grade 2 view, and intubation was successful. Significant hypertrophy of the lingual tonsils was noted. How should airway management be approached during the remainder of perioperative care?

Suggested Answer

A video laryngoscope should remain readily available during the procedure, extubation, and recovery. The report to the surgical team and recovery room staff should include a detailed account of mask ventilation and intubation attempts. The anesthesiologist should document the presence and nature of the airway difficulty in the medical record, including a description of the various airway management techniques that were used. The patient should be informed of his difficult intubation status. Notification systems, such as a written report or letter to the patient, communication with the patient's primary care provider, or a notification bracelet or equivalent identification device may be considered.

References

1. Peterson GN, Domino KB, Caplan RA, Posner KL, Lee LA, Cheney FW. Management of the difficult airway: a closed claims analysis. *Anesthesiology*. 2005 Jul;103(1):33–9.
2. Caplan RA, Benumof JL, Berry FA, et al. Practice guidelines for management of the difficult airway: a report by the American Society of Anesthesiologists Task Force on Management of the Difficult Airway. *Anesthesiology*. 1993; 78:597–602
3. Mort TC. Emergency tracheal intubation: complications associated with repeated laryngoscopic attempts. *Anesth Analg*. 2004 Aug;99(2):607–13.
4. Apfelbaum JL, Hagberg CA, Caplan RA, et al. Practice guidelines for management of the difficult airway: an updated report by the American Society of Anesthesiologists Task Force on Management of the Difficult Airway. *Anesthesiology*. 2013 Feb;118(2):251–70.

3

Predictive Factors of Difficult and Impossible Mask Ventilation

> Given that mask ventilation is an important rescue technique in cases of difficult intubation, the inability to mask ventilate represents an event with significant potential morbidity and mortality.
>
> —KHETERPAL ET AL.[1]

Research Question: What are the incidence and predictors of difficult and impossible mask ventilation (MV) and how do they compare with final airway outcomes?

Year Study Published: 2006.

Study Location: University of Michigan, Ann Arbor, Michigan.

Who Was Studied: Adult patients undergoing general anesthesia over a 24-month period in whom MV was attempted.

Who Was Excluded: Two cases of impossible MV due to an existing patent tracheostomy site.

How Many Patients: 22,660.

Study Overview: See Figure 3.1 for an overview of the study's design.

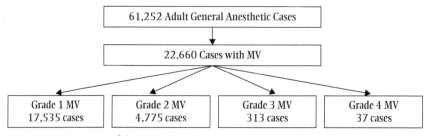

Figure 3.1 Summary of the study design.

Endpoints: Primary outcome: ease or difficulty of MV assessed using a four-point scale ranging from grade 1 to 4 originally described by Han et al.[2] Secondary outcomes: direct laryngoscopy (DL) view as defined by Cormack and Lehane[3], a subjective assessment of difficult intubation due to grade III or IV DL view or more than three intubation attempts, and the ability to perform successful tracheal intubation using DL.

RESULTS

- During the 24-month study period, 22,660 cases of MV attempts were analyzed.
- Three hundred thirteen cases (1.4%) of grade 3 MV (difficult MV), 37 cases (0.16%) of grade 4 MV (impossible MV), and 84 cases (0.37%) of grade 3 or 4 MV in conjunction with difficult intubation were reported (Table 3.1).
- Predictors of grade 3 MV (difficult MV): body mass index (BMI) ≥30 kg/m², age ≥57 years, presence of a beard, Mallampati III or IV, severely limited mandibular protrusion, and snoring.
- Predictors of grade 4 MV (impossible MV): thyromental distance <6 cm and snoring.
- Predictors of grade 3 or 4 MV in conjunction with difficult intubation: limited or severely limited mandibular protrusion, thick/obese neck anatomy, sleep apnea, BMI ≥30 kg/m2, and snoring,
- Of the 37 cases of grade 4 MV (impossible MV), 26 patients were intubated without difficulty, 10 patients were a difficult intubation, and 1 patient could not be intubated and required emergent cricothyrotomy.
- Out of concern for impossible ventilation and intubation, the anesthesia provider may have chosen elective awake fiberoptic intubation, thereby excluding patients from the data set; analysis of patients undergoing

elective awake fiberoptic intubation showed statistically higher rates of risk factors for grade 3 or 4 MV than the standard induction population in the study.

Table 3.1. Mask Ventilation Scale and Incidence

Grade	Description	n (%)
1	Ventilated by mask	17,535 (77.4)
2	Ventilated by mask with oral airway/adjuvant with or without muscle relaxant	4,775 (21.1)
3	Difficult mask ventilation: inadequate to maintain oxygenation, unstable, or requiring two providers, with or without muscle relaxant	313 (1.4)
4	Impossible mask ventilation: unable to mask ventilate with or without muscle relaxant, defined by the absence of end-tidal carbon dioxide measurement and lack of perceptible chest wall movement during positive pressure ventilation attempts despite airway adjuvants and additional personnel	37 (0.16)

Criticisms and Limitations: To avoid interfering with clinical care delivery, the authors did not attempt to standardize conditions across MV and DL attempts, potentially confounding the results. A distinct data collection form with diagrams and extensive definitions to assist providers in accurate selection and documentation was not used. Historically, only three categories of MV had been used (easy, difficult, and impossible), but a more stringent definition of difficult MV was employed in this study, possibly underestimating clinically significant grade 3 MV as a result. With only 37 cases of grade 4 MV observed, the analysis and ability to derive reliable predictors of grade 4 MV are limited by the rarity of the event.

Other Relevant Studies and Information:

- In 2013, Kheterpal et al.[3] published data from the Multicenter Perioperative Outcomes Group on the incidence, predictors, and outcomes of difficult MV combined with difficult laryngoscopy. Six hundred ninety-eight patients experienced grade 3 or 4 MV with difficult laryngoscopy (grade 3 or 4 view or four or more intubation attempts), with an incidence of 0.40% (similar to the 0.37% reported in the 2006 paper).
- In the 2013 report, independent predictors of difficult MV and difficult laryngoscopy included age ≥46 years, BMI ≥30, male gender,

Mallampati III or IV, neck mass or radiation, limited thyromental distance, sleep apnea, presence of teeth, beard, thick neck, limited cervical spine mobility, and limited jaw protrusion.

Summary and Implications: This study was the first to document the incidence and predictors of impossible MV. In this analysis, the incidence of impossible MV was 0.16%. Risk factors for difficult or impossible MV included BMI ≥ 30 kg/m^2, age ≥ 57 years, presence of a beard, Mallampati III or IV, severely limited mandibular protrusion, snoring, and thyromental distance <6 cm. Many of those risk factors, as well as thick/obese neck anatomy and sleep apnea, were also risk factors for difficulty with intubation. Both this and subsequent studies have demonstrated that the overwhelming majority of cases of difficult or impossible MV and difficult intubation are eventually successfully intubated.

CLINICAL CASE: PREPARING FOR DIFFICULT MASK VENTILATION

Case History

A 64-year-old man is evaluated in the preoperative holding area before general anesthesia for a partial colectomy. He is obese with a BMI of 34 kg/m^2 and has not undergone a formal sleep study. He reports heavy snoring with daytime fatigue and is otherwise healthy aside from a colon adenocarcinoma. Airway examination demonstrates a short and thick neck, full range of neck mobility, thyromental distance >6 cm, Mallampati III, normal dentition, normal mandibular protrusion, and the presence of a beard. Based on the preoperative history and examination, how should this patient's airway be managed?

Suggested Answer

This patient demonstrates multiple risk factors for difficult MV. The only easily modifiable risk factor is the presence of a beard, which the patient could be asked to trim. Preparation before induction for MV could include recruiting another anesthesia provider for assistance and having oral, nasal, and laryngeal mask airways readily available. This patient also demonstrates multiple risk factors for difficult intubation. Additional intubation equipment such as a video laryngoscope may be needed and should also be readily available.

References

1. Kheterpal S, Han R, Tremper KK, et al. Incidence and predictors of difficult and impossible mask ventilation. *Anesthesiology* 2006 Nov;105(5):885–91.
2. Han R, Tremper KK, Kheterpal S, O'Reilly M. Grading scale for mask ventilation. *Anesthesiology* 2004 Jul;101(1):267
3. Cormack RS, Lehane J. Difficult tracheal intubation in obstetrics. *Anaesthesia* 1984 Nov;39(11):1105–11
4. Kheterpal S, Healy D, Aziz MF, et al. Incidence, predictors, and outcome of difficult mask ventilation combined with difficult laryngoscopy: a report from the Multicenter Perioperative Outcomes Group. *Anesthesiology* 2013 Dec;119(6):1360–69.

4

Perioperative Normothermia and Incidence of Cardiac Events

In patients with cardiac risk factors who are undergoing noncardiac surgery, the perioperative maintenance of normothermia is associated with a reduced incidence of morbid cardiac events and ventricular tachycardia.

—Frank et al.[1]

Research Question: Does maintenance of perioperative normothermia with supplemental warming reduce the incidence of postoperative cardiac events?

Funding: National Institutes of Health and Mallinckrodt Medical Inc.

Year Study Began: 1992.

Year Study Published: 1997.

Study Location: The Johns Hopkins Hospital.

Who Was Studied: Patients >60 years of age scheduled for peripheral vascular, abdominal, or thoracic surgical procedures with planned postoperative admission to the intensive care unit (ICU). Patients were required either to have a documented history of coronary artery disease or to be considered at high risk for coronary artery disease by established criteria.

Who Was Excluded: Patients with preoperative tympanic temperatures <36° C or >38° C, baseline electrocardiogram abnormalities that interfered with monitoring for ischemia, or a history of Raynaud disease or thyroid disorders.

How Many Patients: 300.

Study Overview: See Figure 4.1 for an overview of the study's design.

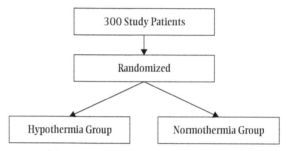

Figure 4.1 Summary of the study design.

Study Intervention: All patients received routine thermal care consisting of the operating room thermostat set to 21° C, warming of all intravenous (IV) fluids and blood products, and passive humidification of the ventilator circuit. For each patient, temperature was monitored at eight locations (two core and six skin-surface sites). Patients in the control (hypothermia) group received either one or two warmed cotton blankets postoperatively, at the nurse's discretion. Patients in the intervention (normothermia) group received an upper body or lower body forced-air warming cover intraoperatively and were treated with a full-body forced-air cover for the first 2 hours of postoperative ICU care.

Follow-Up: 24 hours after surgery.

Endpoints: Primary outcome: morbid cardiac event (cardiac arrest, myocardial infarction, or unstable angina/ischemia). Secondary outcome: Holter monitor–documented ventricular tachycardia (5 or more consecutive wide complex beats at a rate greater than 100 beats per minute).

RESULTS

- Hypothermic and normothermic groups were similar with regard to preoperative demographic variables, anesthetic technique, invasive hemodynamic monitoring, intraoperative blood and fluid requirements, incidence of intraoperative myocardial ischemia or ventricular tachycardia, and incidence of postoperative death.
- Postoperatively, patients in the hypothermia group had more vasoconstriction (increased forearm to fingertip skin-surface temperature gradient), higher incidence of shivering ($P < 0.001$), greater number of hours with hypertension (systolic upper limit prospectively defined, $P = 0.04$) and lower mean core ICU admission temperatures by $1.3°$ C ($P < 0.001$) compared with those in the normothermia group.
- Postoperatively, fewer morbid cardiac events occurred in the normothermic group than in the hypothermic group (1.4% vs. 6.3%; $P = 0.02$).
- Postoperatively, ventricular tachycardia occurred less frequently in the normothermic group than in the hypothermic group (2.4% vs. 7.9%; $P = 0.04$).
- By multivariate analysis, hypothermia was an independent predictor of morbid cardiac events (relative risk = 2.2; 95% confidence interval = 1.1–4.7; $P = 0.04$), indicating a 55% reduction in risk when normothermia was maintained.
- Compared with patients without morbid cardiac events, mean core temperature immediately after surgery was $1°$ C lower for patients with morbid cardiac events. Additionally, median length of ICU stay was 5.5 hours longer for patients suffering morbid cardiac events than for those without events ($P = 0.002$).

Criticisms and Limitations: The incidence of morbid cardiac events was low (12 patients total, 10 in the hypothermic group, and 2 in the normothermic group), limiting the power of the study to assess the impact of normothermia vs. hypothermia on cardiovascular outcomes. The majority of postoperative ventricular tachycardia episodes occurred without symptoms and were deemed to not be clinically significant.

Other Relevant Studies and Information:

- Perioperative hypothermia has also been shown to be associated with increases in surgical bleeding,[2] wound infection, and hospital length of stay.[3]
- The American Society of Anesthesiologists (ASA) Standards for Basic Anesthetic Monitoring state that "every patient receiving anesthesia shall have temperature monitored when clinically significant changes in body temperature are intended, anticipated, or suspected."[4] The ASA Practice Guidelines for Postanesthetic Care state that "patient temperature should be periodically assessed during emergence and recovery."[5]

Summary and Implications: This was the first prospective, randomized controlled trial to examine the relationship between body temperature and cardiac outcomes in the perioperative period. It determined that maintenance of normothermia reduces perioperative cardiac morbidity. Maintenance of perioperative normothermia has become the standard of care.

CLINICAL CASE: PERIOPERATIVE TEMPERATURE MANAGEMENT

Case History

An 88-year-old man with coronary artery disease, hypertension, and peripheral vascular disease presents for thoracotomy and right upper lobe resection for lung cancer. He was a long-term smoker and has multiple coronary artery stents. Given the patient's past medical history and planned surgical procedure, how should this patient be managed in order to maintain perioperative normothermia?

Suggested Answer

A thoracotomy requires significant surgical exposure with potential hypothermia. This patient should be warmed in the preoperative holding area. Intraoperatively, core body temperature should be monitored and maintained by warming IV fluids and blood products, using a heat-moisture exchanger for the ventilator circuit, and placing forced-air blankets both above and below the surgical field if possible. Surgical irrigation fluid should be warmed. The operating room thermostat temperature should be increased if the patient develops hypothermia. Warming should continue in the immediate postoperative period, and the patient's cardiovascular status should be closely monitored.

References

1. Frank SM, Fleisher LA, Breslow MJ, et al. Perioperative maintenance of normothermia reduces the incidence of morbid cardiac events. A randomized clinical trial. *JAMA*. 1997 Apr 9;277(14):1127–34.
2. Schmied H, Kurz A, Sessler DI, Kozek S, Reiter A. Mild hypothermia increases blood loss and transfusion requirements during total hip arthroplasty. *Lancet*. 1996;347:289–92.
3. Kurz A, Sessler DI, Lenhardt R. Perioperative normothermia to reduce the incidence of surgical-wound infection and shorten hospitalization. *N Engl J Med*. 1996;334:1209–15.
4. Standards for Basic Anesthesia Monitoring. ASA website. http://www.asahq.org/quality-and-practice-management/standards-and-guidelines. Approved by the ASA House of Delegates on October 21, 1986, last amended on October 20, 2010, and last affirmed on October 28, 2015. Accessed August 2017.
5. Apfelbaum JL, Silverstein JH, Chung FF, et al. Practice guidelines for postanesthetic care: an updated report by the American Society of Anesthesiologists Task Force on Postanesthetic Care. *Anesthesiology*. 2013 Feb;118(2):291–307.

5

Perioperative Normothermia, Incidence of Surgical-Wound Infection and Length of Hospitalization

Hypothermia itself may delay healing and predispose patients to wound infections. Maintaining normothermia intraoperatively is likely to decrease the incidence of infectious complications in patients undergoing colorectal resection and to shorten their hospitalizations.

—KURZ ET AL.[1]

Research Question: Does perioperative hypothermia increase susceptibility to surgical-wound infection and lengthen hospitalization?

Funding: National Institutes of Health, Joseph Drown and Max Kade Foundations, and Augustine Medical, Inc.

Year Study Began: 1993.

Year Study Published: 1996.

Study Location: University of California, San Francisco and University of Vienna, Vienna, Austria.

Who Was Studied: Patients 18 to 80 years old who underwent elective colo-rectal resection for cancer or inflammatory bowel disease.

Who Was Excluded: Patients undergoing minor colon surgery and those who used immunosuppressive medication during the 4 weeks before surgery; had a recent history of fever, infection, or both; had serious malnutrition (serum albumin <3.3g/dL, white blood cell count <2500 cells/mL, loss of >20% body weight); or had bowel obstruction.

How Many Patients: 200.

Study Overview: See Figure 5.1 for an overview of the study's design.

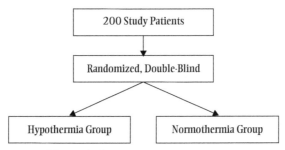

Figure 5.1 Summary of the study design.

Study Intervention: All patients received standardized anesthetic care and perioperative antibiotics. Patients were randomly assigned to routine intraoperative thermal care (the hypothermia group) or additional warming (the normothermia group). Both groups used an intravenous fluid warmer and upper body forced-air cover; the fluid warmer was activated only for patients assigned to the normothermia group, and the forced-air cover was set to ambient temperature for the hypothermia group and at 40° C for the normothermia group. Core and skin temperatures were recorded preoperatively, intraoperatively, and postoperatively. Neither the surgeons nor the patients (double-blind) were informed of their group assignments. Lowest allowable core temperature was 34.5° C for the hypothermia group. Temperatures were not controlled postoperatively.

Follow-Up: 2 weeks postoperatively.

Endpoints: Primary outcome: incidence of surgical wound infections (as defined by the presence of pus and a positive culture diagnosed within 15 days of surgery). Secondary outcomes: duration of hospitalization, days to first solid food, days to suture removal, collagen deposition, vasoconstriction, shivering, and thermal comfort.

RESULTS

- The study was stopped after enrolling 200 patients (intended to include 400 patients) because the difference in incidence of surgical-wound infection between the two study groups reached statistical significance.
- The hypothermia and normothermia groups were similar with regard to preoperative patient demographics, surgical variables (procedure, duration), type of anesthesia, and hemodynamic variables.
- The normothermia group exhibited greater mean (± SD) core body temperatures at end of surgery (36.6° ± 0.5° C vs. 34.7° ± 0.6° C; $P < 0.001$), greater thermal comfort, less shivering, and less vasoconstriction.
- The hypothermia group had three times as many surgical-wound infections as the normothermia group (19% vs. 6%; $P = 0.009$).
- For the hypothermia group, duration of hospitalization was prolonged by 2 days, suture removal and progression to solid food occurred 1 day later, and surgical wounds demonstrated significantly less collagen deposition (Table 5.1). These differences remained significant even if analysis was limited to uninfected patients.
- The hypothermia group required significantly more allogeneic blood transfusions, but transfusion requirement did not independently contribute to the incidence of surgical-wound infection on multivariate regression analysis.
- White blood cell count was significantly lower on the first postoperative day and higher on the third postoperative day in the hypothermia group compared with the normothermia group.
- Patients who smoked had three times as many surgical-wound infections and longer hospitalizations than nonsmokers.

Table 5.1. SUMMARY OF KEY FINDINGS*

Outcome	Normothermia (N = 104)	Hypothermia (N = 96)	P Value
Infection—no. of patients (%)	6 (6)	18 (19)	0.009
Collagen deposition (mg/cm)	328 ± 135	254 ± 114	0.04
Days to first solid food	5.6 ± 2.5	6.5 ± 2	0.006
Days to suture removal	9.8 ± 2.9	10.9 ± 1.9	0.002
Days of hospitalization	12.1 ± 4.4	14.7 ± 6.5	0.001

*Plus-minus values are mean ± SD.

Criticisms and Limitations: This study demonstrated a higher incidence of surgical-wound infection compared with prior reports, possibly because all wounds draining pus that yielded a positive culture were considered infected; the clinical significance of these infections is not known. This study was conducted in Austria, where administrative and cost factors likely do not influence the length of hospital stay to the extent that they might in a managed-care situation.

Other Relevant Studies and Information:

- Surgical-site infections (SSIs) occur in approximately 2%–5% of patients undergoing surgery in the acute care setting in the United States and are associated with increases in length of hospital stay, risk for death, and cost of care.[2] A meta-analysis of studies reporting outcomes of intraoperative hypothermia concluded that hypothermic patients had increased hospitalization costs and adverse outcomes, including a 64% increase in SSIs.[3]
- The incidence of SSI is used as a measure of quality in the clinical setting. Initiated by the Centers for Medicare and Medicaid Services (CMS) and the Centers for Disease Control and Prevention (CDC), the Surgical Care Improvement Project (SCIP) aims to reduce the incidence of surgical complications, including SSIs.[4]
- A randomized controlled trial of clean surgeries (breast, varicose veins, or hernias) found that warming patients for 30 minutes preoperatively reduced infection rates from 14% to 5%.[5]
- In addition to SSIs, intraoperative hypothermia has been associated with various complications, including postoperative cardiac events, increased intraoperative blood loss and transfusion requirements, and increased time to recovery from anesthesia.[6]
- The 2017 CDC Guideline for the Prevention of Surgical Site Infection states that perioperative normothermia should be maintained. (Category IA–strong recommendation; high to moderate–quality evidence.)[7]

Summary and Implications: This trial demonstrated that perioperative hypothermia during major surgery increases the incidence of surgical-wound infection, lengthens hospitalization, and adversely affects additional outcomes, including collagen formation, days to first solid food, and days to suture removal. Guidelines now recommend the use of warming devices and temperature monitoring to reduce the rate of perioperative hypothermia.

CLINICAL CASE: PERIOPERATIVE TEMPERATURE MANAGEMENT

Case History

A small community hospital has seven operating rooms but only three fluid warmers and three forced-air warmers. The latest analysis of the hospital's outcome data demonstrated an increased rate of SSIs in colorectal surgery patients compared with the national average. Should additional warming devices be purchased and their use standardized for colorectal procedures?

Suggested Answer

Perioperative hypothermia increases the incidence of adverse events, length of hospitalization, and cost of care. In considering the benefits of maintaining normothermia, it is important to consider the number and types of surgical procedures being performed. If a small hospital performs a substantial number of procedures of short duration under monitored anesthesia care or regional block, then purchasing additional warming devices may not offer additional benefit. Analyzing the hospital's perioperative temperature data, particularly for patients undergoing colorectal procedures, may yield additional insight.

References

1. Kurz A, Sessler DI, Lenhardt R. Perioperative normothermia to reduce the incidence of surgical-wound infection and shorten hospitalization. *N Engl J Med.* 1996;334:1209–1215.
2. Beltramini AM, Salata RA, Ray AJ. Thermoregulation and risk of surgical site infection. *Infect Control Hosp Epidemiol.* 2011 Jun;32(6):603–10.
3. Mahoney CB, Odom J. Maintaining intraoperative normothermia: a meta-analysis of outcomes with costs. *AANA J.* 1999 Apr;67(2):155–63.
4. Rosenberger LH, Politano AD, Sawyer RG. The surgical care improvement project and prevention of post-operative infection, including surgical site infection. *Surg Infect (Larchmt).* 2011 Jun;12(3):163–68.
5. Melling AC, Ali B, Scott EM, Leaper DJ. Effects of preoperative warming on the incidence of wound infection after clean surgery: a randomised controlled trial. *Lancet.* 2001 Sep 15;358(9285):876–80.
6. Reynolds L, Beckmann J, Kurz A. Perioperative complications of hypothermia. *Best Pract Res Clin Anaesthesiol.* 2008 Dec;22(4):645–57.
7. Berrios-Torres SI, Umscheid CA, Bratzler DW et al. Centers for Disease Control and Prevention Guideline for the Prevention of Surgical Site Infection, 2017. *JAMA Surg.* 2017 Aug 1;152(8):784–91.

6

Preventable Anesthesia Mishaps

A modified critical-incident analysis technique was used in a retro-spective examination of the characteristics of human error and equip-ment failure in anesthetic practice. Most of the preventable incidents involved human error (82%), with breathing-circuit disconnections, inadvertent changes in gas flow, and drug syringe errors being frequent problems.

—COOPER ET AL.[1]

Research Question: How does human error contribute to preventable anes-thesia mishaps, and are there patterns in frequently occurring incidents that need prospective investigation and prevention measures?

Funding: National Institute of General Medical Sciences.

Year Study Began: 1975.

Year Study Published: 1978.

Study Location: Massachusetts General Hospital, Boston, Massachusetts.

Who Was Studied: Anesthesia personnel (residents and attendings) were asked to describe mishaps that they observed or were directly involved in at any point in their professional careers. A mishap was labeled a critical incident when it was an occurrence that could have led or did lead to an undesirable outcome. Incidents were required to have the following characteristics: (1) involved an error by a member of the anesthesia team or a failure of the anesthetist's equipment to function properly; (2) occurred at a time when the patient was under the care of an anesthetist; (3) was described in clear detail by a person who either observed or was involved in the incident; (4) was clearly preventable.

Who Was Excluded: Incidents were excluded when doubt existed about preventability, as assessed by the anesthesia personnel.

How Many Patients: A total of 47 interviews were conducted, and descriptions of 359 preventable incidents were obtained.

Study Overview: See Figure 6.1 for an overview of the study's design.

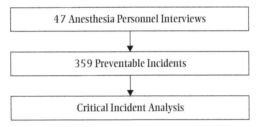

Figure 6.1 Summary of the study design.

Study Intervention: A series of 25 pilot interviews were conducted to evaluate interview strategies and develop an interview format. Information collected during pilot interviews was used to develop an initial incident classification scheme. Study interviewees were selected at random and introduced to the study by a brief letter. All interviews were conducted by the same interviewer and lasted 60 to 90 minutes. Incident details were coded using a branching classification scheme with 23 major categories of information.

Endpoints: Computer-aided analysis for trends and patterns of the database. The data were examined by generating summaries of the 23 major categories of information and by numerical sorting techniques in search for nonobvious cluster of incident types and surrounding circumstances.

RESULTS

- A total of 359 preventable incidents were identified and coded, of which 55% had occurred within 1 year before the interview, 82% involved human error, and 14% involved equipment failure.
- Staff averaged seven incidents per interview; residents averaged eight incidents per interview.
- The seriousness of the incidents ranged from events that had no known negative effects to the patient to incidents that resulted in patient death.
- The 10 categories of most frequently occurring incidents are listed in Table 6.1.
- Critical incidents occurred most commonly during the middle of the anesthetic and frequently during the induction period.
- A subset of incidents involved the relief of one anesthetist by another. In most cases, the relieving anesthetist identified a problem, suggesting that a policy of periodic breaks is preferred to such breaks not being permitted.
- A category of "associated factors" was developed in response to information collected during the interviews, and these factors were believed to be predisposing circumstances associated with the incidents (Table 6.2).

Table 6.1. THE MOST FREQUENTLY OCCURRING INCIDENTS

Incident	Number of Occurrences
Breathing circuit disconnection	27
Inadvertent gas flow change	22
Syringe swap	19
Gas supply problem	15
Intravenous apparatus disconnection	11
Laryngoscope malfunction	11
Premature extubation	10
Breathing circuit connection error	9
Hypovolemia	9
Tracheal airway device position change	7

Table 6.2. SUMMARY OF ASSOCIATED FACTORS CITED

Associated Factor	Number of Occurrences
Inadequate total experience	77
Inadequate familiarity with equipment/device	45
Poor communication with team, lab, etc.	27
Haste	26
Inattention/carelessness	26
Fatigue	24
Excessive dependency on other personnel	24
Failure to perform a normal check	22
Training or experience—other factors	22
Supervisor not present enough	18
Environmental or colleagues—other factors	18
Visual field restricted	17
Mental or physical—other factors	16
Inadequate familiarity with surgical procedure	14
Distraction	13
Poor labeling of controls, drugs, etc.	12
Supervision—other factors	12
Situation precluded normal precautions	10
Inadequate familiarity with anesthetic technique	10
Teaching activity underway	9
Apprehension	8
Emergency case	6
Demanding or difficult case	6
Boredom	5
Nature of activity—other factors	5
Insufficient preparation	3
Slow procedure	3
Other	3

Criticisms and Limitations: This retrospective examination of critical incidents relied on anesthesia providers to recall information from the remote past. All incidents that involved breathing circuit disconnections were arbitrarily treated as human error; because the frequency of such disconnections is a direct consequence of equipment design, these incidents could alternatively be considered equipment failures. Information regarding the time of day that an incident occurred (day vs. night) was deliberately elicited during only the final 19 interviews.

Other Relevant Studies and Information:

- A follow-up study involving four hospitals was reported in 1984 that included a more detailed analysis and 10 potential strategies for prevention or detection of critical incidents.[2]
- A recent analysis of the American Society of Anesthesiologists Closed Claims database showed that for claims from 1990 to 2007, the leading outcomes were death (26%), nerve injury (22%), and permanent brain damage (9%). The most common damaging events due to anesthesia in claims were regional-block–related (20%), respiratory (17%), cardiovascular (13%) and equipment-related events (10%).[3]
- A study published in 2015 used a voluntary critical incident reporting system to identify opportunities to improve clinical care and patient safety. A 20-item list of complications was completed for each procedure, and all critical incidents were entered into an anesthesia information management system and reclassified into 95 different critical incidents. During the 110,310 procedures performed, 3904 critical incidents in 3807 (3.5%) anesthetic procedures were identified. Technical difficulties with regional anesthesia ($n = 445$; 40 per 10,000 anesthetics), hypotension ($n = 432$; 39 per 10,000 anesthetics), and unexpected difficult intubation ($n = 216$; 20 per 10,000 anesthetics) were the most frequently documented critical incidents.[4]

Summary and Implications: This study established a framework for assessing patient safety in anesthesiology and exposed patterns of frequently occurring preventable incidents. These data also suggested that the application of human-factors principles could be used in anesthesia, following the example of success in fields such as aviation.

CLINICAL CASE: FLUID RESUSCITATION IN THE INTENSIVE CARE UNIT

Case History

A 27-year-old woman underwent an elective cesarean delivery under spinal anesthesia. After the baby was delivered, the patient experienced severe nausea. The anesthesia provider intended to administer ondansetron but inadvertently administered undiluted phenylephrine. The patient complained of a headache and became hypertensive. Nitroglycerine was administered with resolution of symptoms. What follow-up for this medication error is necessary?

Suggested Answer

After the patient has recovered from anesthesia, a disclosure of the adverse event should be made and documented. The medication error should be reported to a quality and safety committee for review.

References

1. Cooper JB, Newbower RS, Long CD, McPeek B. Preventable anesthesia mishaps: a study of human factors. *Anesthesiology.* 1978 Dec;49(6):399–406.
2. Cooper JB, Newbower RS, Kitz RJ. An analysis of major errors and equipment failures in anesthesia management: considerations for prevention and detection. *Anesthesiology.* 1984 Jan;60(1):34–42.
3. Metzner J, Posner KL, Lam MS, Domino KB. Closed claims' analysis. *Best Pract Res Clin Anaesthesiol.* 2011 Jun;25(2):263–76.
4. Munting KE, van Zaane B, Schouten AN, van Wolfswinkel L, de Graaff JC. Reporting critical incidents in a tertiary hospital: a historical cohort study of 110,310 procedures. *Can J Anaesth.* 2015 Dec;62(12):1248–58.

7

Deliberate Increase of Oxygen Delivery in the Perioperative Period

Perioperative increase of oxygen delivery with dopexamine hydrochloride significantly reduces mortality and morbidity in high-risk surgical patients.

—BOYD ET AL.[1]

Research Question: Does the deliberate increase in oxygen delivery with the use of perioperative dopexamine reduce mortality and morbidity in high-risk surgical patients?

Funding: Fisons, PLC, United Kingdom.

Year Study Began: 1990.

Year Study Published: 1993.

Study Location: St. George's Hospital, London, England.

Who Was Studied: Patients undergoing surgery expecting to last or lasting more than 1.5 hours who were identified as high risk by the following: previous severe cardiorespiratory illness, extensive surgery planned for carcinoma, acute blood loss >8 units, age >70 years with limited physiologic reserve in one or more organs, respiratory failure, acute abdominal catastrophe with hemodynamic instability, acute renal failure, and late-state vascular disease involving aortic disease.

How Many Patients: 107.

Study Overview: See Figure 7.1 for an overview of the study's design.

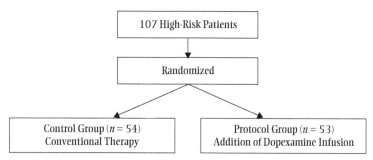

Figure 7.1 Summary of the study design.

Study Intervention: Dopexamine is a dopamine analogue that produces peripheral vasodilation and an increase in cardiac index without significant increases in myocardial oxygen consumption. High-risk surgical patients were randomized to control or protocol limbs of the study. Patients in both groups had arterial and pulmonary artery catheters placed. Preoperatively, all patients were optimized in accordance with identical treatment goals, including mean arterial pressure 80–110 mm Hg; pulmonary artery occlusion pressure 12–14 mm Hg; arterial oxygen saturation >94%; hemoglobin >12 g/dL; and urine output >0.5 mL/kg/h.

Patients randomized to the dopexamine group were further treated with the study drug if oxygen delivery (DO_2I) had not reached 600 mL/min/m². Dopexamine was infused starting at a dose of 0.5 µg/kg/min and was doubled every 30 minutes to a maximum dose of 8 µg/kg/min or until a DO_2I of 600 mL/min/m² was achieved. Further increases in dopexamine dose were limited if patients experienced chest pain, significant ST depression on electrocardiogram, or an increase in heart rate greater than 20% from baseline. Intraoperatively, dopexamine was continued at the infusion dose reached preoperatively.

Postoperatively, additional qualifying patients identified during surgery were likewise randomized to control or protocol limbs of the study and had pulmonary artery catheters inserted and treatment instituted within 2 hours of the end of surgery. Postoperatively, the same treatment goals and dopexamine dosing regimen as used preoperatively were maintained. There were no restrictions placed on intraoperative or postoperative management. DO_2I was calculated as: DO_2I (mL/min/m²) = CI (L/min/m²) × Sao_2 (%) × Hb (g/L) × 0.0134.

Follow-up: 28 days postoperatively.

Endpoints: Mortality and complications (respiratory failure, acute renal failure, sepsis, cardiorespiratory arrest, pulmonary edema, pleural fluid, wound infection, disseminated intravascular coagulation, acute myocardial infarction, abdominal abscess, postoperative hemorrhage, gastric outlet obstruction, cerebrovascular accident, pulmonary embolism, chest infection, psychosis, distal ischemia, and other).

RESULTS

- There were no significant differences between the two study groups with regard to demographic characteristics, known surgical risk factors (e.g., smoking, diabetes), study admission criteria, or proportion of emergency or urgent surgical procedures.
- Patients in the dopexamine group had significantly higher oxygen delivery indices preoperatively and postoperatively.
- Oxygen consumption was not significantly different between the two study groups.
- Patients in the dopexamine group received significantly more fluid preoperatively than the control group ($P < 0.01$), but there was no significant difference in postoperative fluid management in the first 24 hours between the two study groups.
- Mortality at 28 days was significantly lower ($P = 0.015$) in the dopexamine group (5.7%) vs. the control group (22.2%), demonstrating a 75% reduction.
- The biggest difference in mortality was observed in abdominal surgery patients.
- The number of complications per patient was significantly lower in the dopexamine group compared with the control group ($P = 0.008$).

Criticisms and Limitations: This study could not be blinded for investigators given that dopexamine infusions were titrated to attain a specific target for oxygen delivery; however, neither the surgeon nor anesthesiologist was aware of a particular patient's study group allocation. Nine patients randomized to the dopexamine group preoperatively were not treated in accordance with the regimen for protocol patients, and all deaths occurring in the dopexamine group were from this group of nine patients (analyses were performed on an intention-to-treat basis). The dopexamine group trended toward shorter intensive care unit and hospital lengths of stay, but the study would have required more than 500 patients to demonstrate a significant difference in length of stay.

Other Relevant Studies and Information:

- In 1960, Clowes and Del Guercio[2] reported that survivors of major operations consistently demonstrated higher postoperative values for cardiac output and oxygen delivery than patients who subsequently died. In 1988, the work of Shoemaker et al.[3] demonstrated reduced mortality and morbidity in high-risk surgical patients when cardiac output and oxygen delivery values became additional goals for perioperative management.
- A 2014 meta-analysis of randomized controlled trials examined whether goal-directed therapy (GDT) using fluid challenges and inotropes to augment oxygen delivery increased the risk for cardiac complications in high-risk, noncardiac surgical patients. Studies that included cardiac, trauma, and pediatric surgeries were excluded. Rates of cardiac complications, arrhythmias, myocardial ischemia, and acute pulmonary edema were examined. GDT was associated with a reduction in total cardiovascular complications ($P = 0.0005$) and arrhythmias ($P = 0.007$). GDT was not associated with an increase in acute pulmonary edema or myocardial ischemia.[4]
- In a 20-year retrospective review[5] of this study by the same authors, they conclude with the statement that they "hope that the concept of goal-directed perioperative therapy for major surgery continues to improve outcomes and becomes the international standard of care."

Summary and Implications: This randomized controlled study demonstrated a significant reduction in mortality and morbidity when dopexamine was used to increase oxygen delivery during the perioperative period in high-risk surgical patients.

References

1. Boyd O, Grounds RM, Bennett ED. A randomized clinical trial of the effect of deliberate perioperative increase of oxygen delivery on mortality in high-risk surgical patients. *JAMA*. 1993 Dec 8;270(22):2699–707.
2. Clowes GHA Jr, Del Guercio LRM. Circulatory response to trauma of surgical operations. *Metabolism*. 1960;9:67–81.

3. Shoemaker WC, Appel PL, Kram HB, Waxman K, Lee TS. Prospective trial of supranormal values of survivors as therapeutic goals in high-risk surgical patients. *Chest*. 1988;94:1176–1186.
4. Arulkumaran N, Corredor C, Hamilton MA, et al. Cardiac complications associated with goal-directed therapy in high-risk surgical patients: a meta-analysis. *Br J Anaesth*. 2014 Apr;112(4):648–59.
5. Boyd O, Grounds RM. Our study 20 years on: a randomized clinical trial of the effect of deliberate perioperative increase of oxygen delivery on mortality in high-risk surgical patients. *Intensive Care Med*. 2013;39:2107–2114.

8

Blood Sugar Control in Type 2 Diabetes

One message that has been pushed down our throats for over twenty years at least is that the lower your blood glucose levels are the better. . . . The surprising results of the [ACCORD trial are] that . . . there were more deaths in the intensive therapy group than in the standard therapy group.
—Dr. David McCulloch

Research Question: Should doctors target a "normal" blood glucose level in patients with type 2 diabetes?[1]

Funding: The National Heart, Lung, and Blood Institute (NHLBI).

Year Study Began: 2001.

Year Study Published: 2008.

Study Location: 77 centers in the United States and Canada.

Who Was Studied: Patients 40–79 years old with type 2 diabetes, a hemoglobin A1c (HbA1c) level ≥7.5%, and known cardiovascular disease or risk factors.

Who Was Excluded: Patients who were unwilling to do home blood glucose monitoring or unwilling to inject insulin; patients with frequent hypoglycemic episodes; and patients with a creatinine >1.5 mg/dL.

How Many Patients: 10,251.

Study Overview: See Figure 8.1 for an overview of the study's design.

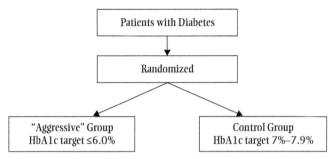

Figure 8.1 Summary of the ACCORD study design.

Study Intervention: Physicians could use any available diabetes medications to achieve the blood glucose targets. Metformin was used in 60% of the patients, insulin in 35%, and sulfonylureas in 50%.

Follow-Up: Mean of 3.5 years.

Endpoints: Primary outcome: a composite of nonfatal myocardial infarction, nonfatal stroke, or death from cardiovascular causes. Secondary outcome: all-cause mortality.

RESULTS

- The mean baseline HbA1c in both groups was 8.1%.
- The mean posttreatment HbA1c in the "aggressive" group was 6.4% vs. 7.5% in the control group.
- The mean weight gain in the "aggressive" group was 3.5 kg vs. 0.4 kg in the control group (Table 8.1).

Table 8.1. SUMMARY OF ACCORD's KEY FINDINGS

Outcome	"Aggressive" Group	Control Group	P Value
Hypoglycemia requiring medical assistance	10.5%	3.5%	<0.001
Cardiovascular events or cardiac death	6.9%	7.2%	0.16
All-cause mortality	5%	4%	0.04

Criticisms and Limitations: The study only included patients with cardio-vascular disease or risk factors and does not provide information about which medications may have been responsible for the excess mortality in the "aggressive group."

Other Relevant Studies and Information:

- The increased mortality rate among patients in the "aggressive" group persisted after 5 years of follow-up.[2]
- Another report involving the ACCORD data showed that, despite the increased mortality, patients in the "aggressive" group had lower rates of early-stage microvascular disease ("albuminuria and some eye complications and neuropathy").[3]
- The Veteran's Affairs Diabetes Trial (VADT) compared "aggressive" blood glucose management (targeting "normal" blood glucose levels) with standard glucose management and found no benefit of the aggressive approach.[4]
- The ADVANCE trial found that patients treated for an HbA1c target of 6.5% had lower rates of diabetes-related complications, primarily nephropathy, than did patients treated for a standard HbA1c target.[5]
- Most clinical practice guidelines recommend an HbA1c target of 6.5%–7.5% and less aggressive targets for patients at high risk for hypoglycemia such as older adults.

Summary and Implications: In the ACCORD trial, a target HbA1c of ≤6.0% was associated with increased mortality compared with a target of 7%–7.9%. Targeting an HbA1c ≤6.0% was associated with reduced early-stage microvascular disease, however. The optimal HbA1c target in patients with diabetes remains an area of active investigation.

CLINICAL CASE: INTENSIVE VS. CONSERVATIVE BLOOD SUGAR CONTROL

Case History

A 60-year-old woman with long-standing type 2 diabetes, hypertension, and hyperlipidemia presents for a routine office visit. Her diabetes medications include metformin 1,000 mg twice daily, insulin glargine 40 units at bedtime, and regular insulin 12 units before each meal. She proudly shows you her blood sugar log, which demonstrates excellent sugar control, with fasting morning sugars averaging 82. Her most recent HbA1c is 6.4%. Her only concerns are her continued inability to lose weight and occasional episodes of "shaking" when her blood sugars drop below 75.

After reading the ACCORD trial, what adjustments might you make to her diabetes medications?

Suggested Answer

The ACCORD trial showed that aggressive blood sugar management with a target HbA1c of ≤6% was associated with increased mortality. In addition, targeting an HbA1c of ≤6% led to weight gain and an increased rate of hypoglycemic episodes. This patient's HbA1c is 6.4%—which was the mean HbA1c level in patients assigned to the "aggressive" blood sugar group in ACCORD. Thus, this patient's blood sugar control is probably too tight, and her insulin dose (either the insulin glargine, regular insulin, or both depending on her blood sugar patterns) should be reduced. This change would be expected to reduce the frequency of her hypoglycemic episodes, make it easier for her to lose weight, and perhaps reduce her risk for death.

References

1. Action to Control Cardiovascular Risk in Diabetes Study Group. Effects of intensive glucose lowering in type 2 diabetes. *N Engl J Med.* 2008;358(24):2545–59.
2. The ACCORD Study Group. Long-term effects of intensive glucose lowering on cardiovascular outcomes. *N Engl J Med.* 2011;364(9):818–28.
3. Ismail-Beigi F, Craven T, Banerji MA, et al. Effect of intensive treatment of hyperglycaemia on microvascular outcomes in type 2 diabetes: an analysis of the ACCORD randomised trial. *Lancet.* 2010;376(9739):419–30.
4. Duckworth W, Abraira C, Moritz T, et al. Glucose control and vascular complications in veterans with type 2 diabetes. *N Engl J Med.* 2009;360(2):129–39.
5. The ADVANCE Collaborative Group. Intensive blood glucose control and vascular outcomes in patients with type 2 diabetes. *N Engl J Med.* 2008;358(24):2560–72.

SECTION 2

Cardiac Anesthesia

Congestive Heart Failure and Pulmonary Artery Catheterization

Addition of the [pulmonary artery catheter] to careful clinical assessment increased anticipated adverse events, but did not affect overall mortality and hospitalization.

—The ESCAPE Investigators[1]

Research Question: Does pulmonary artery catheter (PAC) use improve clinical outcomes in patients hospitalized with severe symptomatic and recurrent heart failure?

Funding: National Heart, Lung, and Blood Institute.

Year Study Began: 2000.

Year Study Published: 2005.

Study Location: 26 heart failure centers in the United States and Canada.

Who Was Studied: Patients with severe symptomatic heart failure with hospitalization for heart failure within the prior year, urgent visit to the emergency department, or treatment during the preceding month with more than 160 mg of furosemide daily (or equivalent). Randomization required at least 3 months of symptoms despite angiotensin-converting enzyme inhibitors and diuretics, ejection fraction ≤30%, systolic blood pressure ≤125 mm Hg, and at least one sign and one symptom of congestion.

Who Was Excluded: Patients with a creatinine level >3.5 mg/dL, prior use of dobutamine or dopamine at >3 μg/kg/min, or use of milrinone during the study hospitalization.

How Many Patients: 433.

Study Overview: See Figure 9.1 for an overview of the study's design.

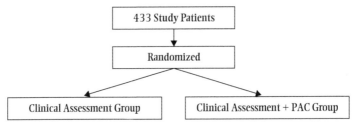

Figure 9.1 Summary of the study design.

Study Intervention: For patients in both study groups, the treatment goal was resolution of clinical signs and symptoms of congestion (jugular venous pressure elevation, edema, orthopnea). For the PAC group, additional treatment goals included reducing pulmonary capillary wedge pressure to ≤15 mm Hg and right atrial pressure to ≤8 mm Hg.

Follow-Up: 6 months.

Endpoints: Primary outcome: days alive out of the hospital during the first 6 months after randomization. Secondary outcome: exercise, quality of life, biochemical markers (natriuretic peptides), and echocardiographic changes.

RESULTS

- The data and safety monitoring board recommended that the trial be stopped before enrolling 500 patients because of concerns of PAC adverse events and the unlikelihood of achieving a significant difference in the primary endpoint.
- Patients in the two randomized groups had similar baseline characteristics.

- The primary endpoint was identical in both groups, and there was no significant difference between subgroups.
- The overall mortality rate was 19% at 6 months. There was no significant difference in the mean number of days patients were well, number of deaths, hospitalizations per patient, or days hospitalized.
- The total number of in-hospital adverse events was significantly higher in the PAC arm of the study (patients with at least one adverse event: 21.9% vs. 11.5%; $P = 0.04$). PAC-related adverse events occurred in a total of 10 patients: PAC-related infection (4 patients), bleeding (2 patients), catheter knotting (2 patients), pulmonary infarction/hemorrhage (2 patients), ventricular tachycardia (1 patient).
- Exercise and quality-of-life endpoints showed greater improvement in the PAC arm.

Criticisms and Limitations: ESCAPE centers were selected for their expertise in treating advanced heart failure patients, and these findings may not be generalizable to other settings. Clinicians were not provided with a standard treatment protocol to implement based on the PAC findings. It is possible that a benefit for PACs might emerge if clinicians used a standardized, evidence-based protocol for responding to the data.

Other Relevant Studies and Information:

- In a secondary analysis of data from ESCAPE by Palardy et al.[2] published in 2009, mitral regurgitation, as assessed by echocardiography, was more effectively reduced when therapy to relieve congestion was guided by PAC goals than by clinical assessment alone during hospitalization. This difference was largely lost after 3 months of outpatient management.
- During the ESCAPE trial, patients who were not randomized because a PAC was considered to be required for management were entered into a concurrent PAC registry. In 2008, Allan et al.[3] published an analysis of 439 PAC registry patients that demonstrated longer hospitalizations (13 vs. 6 days, $P < 0.001$) and higher 6-month mortality (34% vs. 20%, $P < 0.001$) than trial patients, highlighting the complex context of patient selection for randomized trials.
- The 2013 guidelines from the American College of Cardiology Foundation/American Heart Association (ACCF/AHA)[4] indicate

that the "routine use of invasive hemodynamic monitoring is not recommended in normotensive patients with acute decompensated heart failure and congestion with symptomatic response to diuretics and vasodilators" (Box 9.1).

BOX 9.1. 2013 ACCF/AHA GUIDELINES FOR PULMONARY ARTERY CATHETER USE

Class I Recommendation

Invasive hemodynamic monitoring with a pulmonary artery catheter should be performed to guide therapy in patients who have respiratory distress or clinical evidence of impaired perfusion in whom the adequacy or excess of intracardiac filling pressures cannot be determined from clinical assessment. (Level of Evidence: C)

Class IIa Recommendation

Invasive hemodynamic monitoring can be useful for carefully selected patients with acute heart failure who have persistent symptoms despite empiric adjustment of standard therapies and (a) whose fluid status, perfusion, or systemic or pulmonary vascular resistance is uncertain; (b) whose systolic pressure remains low, or is associated with symptoms, despite initial therapy; (c) whose renal function is worsening with therapy; (d) who require parenteral vasoactive agents; or (e) who may need consideration for mechanical circulatory support or transplantation. (Level of Evidence: C)

Class III Recommendation: No Benefit

Routine use of invasive hemodynamic monitoring is not recommended in normotensive patients with acute decompensated heart failure and congestion with symptomatic response to diuretics and vasodilators. (Level of Evidence: B)

Summary and Implications: The ESCAPE trial was the first large, multicenter, randomized clinical trial designed to evaluate the use of PAC in heart failure patients. The trial failed to demonstrate a benefit of PACs. PACs are no longer recommended for guiding the management of patients with heart failure in the intensive care unit setting.

CLINICAL CASE: PULMONARY ARTERY CATHETER USE IN MANAGING HEART FAILURE

Case History
A 59-year-old man is admitted for management of recurrent acute decompensated heart failure. The patient reports weight gain, lower extremity swelling, and decreased functional status for approximately 2 weeks. The patient is normotensive. Is insertion of a PAC in this patient indicated?

Suggested Answer
Standard therapy with diuretics and vasodilators should be implemented. If the patient has persistent symptoms despite adjustments in standard therapy as well as findings such as worsening renal function or requirement for parenteral vasoactive agents, insertion of a PAC for invasive hemodynamic monitoring may be considered.

References

1. Binanay C, Califf RM, Hasselblad V, et al. Evaluation study of congestive heart failure and pulmonary artery catheterization effectiveness: the ESCAPE trial. *JAMA*. 2005 Oct 5;294(13):1625–33.
2. Palardy M, Stevenson LW, Tasissa G, et al. Reduction in mitral regurgitation during therapy guided by measured filling pressures in the ESCAPE trial. *Circ Heart Fail*. 2009 May;2(3):181–8.
3. Allen LA, Rogers JG, Warnica JW, et al. High mortality without ESCAPE: the registry of heart failure patients receiving pulmonary artery catheters without randomization. *J Card Fail*. 2008 Oct;14(8):661–69.
4. Yancy CW, Jessup M, Bozkurt B, et al. 2013 ACCF/AHA guideline for the management of heart failure: a report of the American College of Cardiology Foundation/ American Heart Association Task Force on Practice Guidelines. *Circulation*. 2013 Oct 15;128(16):e240–327.

10

Rate Control vs. Rhythm Control
for Atrial Fibrillation

[In older patients with atrial fibrillation and cardiovascular risk factors]
the strategy of restoring and maintaining sinus rhythm [has] no clear advantage over the strategy of controlling the ventricular rate.
—THE AFFIRM INVESTIGATORS[1]

Research Question: Should patients with atrial fibrillation be managed with a
strategy of rate control or rhythm control?[1]

Funding: The National Heart, Lung, and Blood Institute.

Year Study Began: 1997.

Year Study Published: 2002.

Study Location: 200 sites in the United States and Canada.

Who Was Studied: Adults with atrial fibrillation who were at least 65 years old
or who had other risk factors for stroke. In addition, only patients likely to have
recurrent atrial fibrillation requiring long-term treatment were eligible.

Who Was Excluded: Patients in whom anticoagulation was contraindicated.

How Many Patients: 4,060.

Study Overview: See Figure 10.1 for an overview of the study's design.

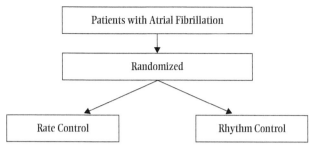

Figure 10.1 Summary of the AFFIRM study design.

Study Intervention: Patients in the rhythm-control group received antiar-rhythmic drugs (most commonly amiodarone and/or sotalol) at the discretion of the treating physician. If needed, physicians could attempt to cardiovert patients to sinus rhythm. Anticoagulation with warfarin was encouraged but could be stopped at the physician's discretion if the patient remained in sinus rhythm for at least 4 (and preferably 12) consecutive weeks.

Patients in the rate-control group received beta blockers, calcium channel blockers, or digoxin at the discretion of the treating physician. The target heart rate was ≤80 beats per minute at rest and ≤110 beats per minute during a 6-minute walk test. All patients in the rate-control group received anticoagulation with warfarin.

Follow-Up: Mean of 3.5 years.

Endpoints: Primary outcome: all-cause mortality. Secondary outcomes: a composite of death, disabling stroke, disabling anoxic encephalopathy, major bleeding, and cardiac arrest and hospitalizations.

RESULTS

- In the rate-control group, at the 5-year visit, 34.6% of patients were in sinus rhythm, and more than 80% of those in atrial fibrillation had adequate heart rate control.
- In the rhythm-control group, at the 5-year visit, 62.6% of patients were in sinus rhythm.
- After 5 years, 14.9% of patients in the rate-control group crossed over to the rhythm-control group, most commonly because of symptoms such as palpitations or episodes of heart failure.
- After 5 years, 37.5% of patients in the rhythm-control group crossed over to the rate-control group, most commonly because of an inability to maintain sinus rhythm or because of drug intolerance.

- Throughout the study, more than 85% of patients in the rate-control group were taking warfarin compared with approximately 70% of patients in the rhythm-control group; most strokes in both groups occurred among patients not receiving a therapeutic dose of warfarin.
- Patients in the rate-control group had fewer hospitalizations than those in the rhythm-control group, and there was a nonsignificant trend toward lower mortality (Table 10.1).

Table 10.1. SUMMARY OF AFFIRM'S KEY FINDINGS

Outcome	Rate-Control Group	Rhythm-Control Group	P Value
All-cause mortality	25.9%	26.7%	0.08
Composite of death, disabling stroke, disabling anoxic encephalopathy, major bleeding, and cardiac arrest	32.7%	32.0%	0.33
Hospitalizations	73.0%	80.1%	<0.001

Criticisms and Limitations: The trial did not include young patients without cardiovascular risk factors, especially those with paroxysmal atrial fibrillation, and therefore the results may not apply to these patients.

In addition, approximately half of the patients in the study had symptomatic episodes of atrial fibrillation less than once a month. It is possible that patients with more frequent or persistent symptoms would derive a benefit from rhythm control.

Other Relevant Studies and Information:

- A number of smaller randomized trials comparing rate control and rhythm control in patients with atrial fibrillation have come to similar conclusions as AFFIRM.[2–5]
- Trials comparing rate control with rhythm control in patients with atrial fibrillation and heart failure have also failed to show a benefit of rhythm control.[6,7]
- A recent observational study suggested lower long-term mortality with a rhythm-control strategy vs. a rate-control strategy.[8] However, because this was not a randomized trial the results are far from definitive and should not lead to a change in clinical practice.[9]

Summary and Implications: In high-risk patients with atrial fibrillation, a strategy of rate control is at least as effective as a strategy of rhythm control. Rhythm control does not appear to obviate the need for anticoagulation. Because the medications used for rate control are usually safer than those used for rhythm control, rate control is the preferred strategy for treating most high-risk patients with atrial fibrillation. These findings do not necessarily apply to younger patients without cardiovascular risk factors who were not included in AFFIRM, however.

CLINICAL CASE: RATE VS. RHYTHM CONTROL IN ATRIAL FIBRILLATION

Case History

A 75-year-old woman with diabetes and hypertension is noted on routine examination to have an irregular heart rate of approximately 120 beats per minute. She denies chest pain, shortness of breath, and other concerning symptoms. An electrocardiogram confirms a diagnosis of atrial fibrillation.

Based on the results of AFFIRM, how should this patient be treated?

Suggested Answer

AFFIRM showed that rate control is at least as effective as rhythm control for managing atrial fibrillation. Because the medications used for rate control are usually safer than those used for rhythm control, rate control is generally the preferred strategy for managing the condition.

The patient in this vignette is typical of patients included in AFFIRM. Thus, she should be treated initially with a rate-control strategy (beta blockers are frequently used as first-line agents). In the unlikely event that this patient's heart rate could not be controlled or if she were to develop bothersome symptoms that did not improve with a rate-control strategy, rhythm control might be considered. In addition, this patient should receive anticoagulation to reduce her risk for stroke.

References

1. The AFFIRM Investigators. A comparison of rate control and rhythm control in patients with atrial fibrillation. *N Engl J Med*. 2002;347(23):1825–33.
2. Van Gelder IC, Hagens VE, Bosker HA, et al. A comparison of rate control and rhythm control in patients with recurrent persistent atrial fibrillation. *N Engl J Med*. 2002;347(23):1834–40.

3. Hohnloser SH, Kuck KH, Lilienthal J. Rhythm or rate control in atrial fibrillation: Pharmacological Intervention in Atrial Fibrillation (PIAF); a randomised trial. *Lancet.* 2000; 356(9244):1789–94.

4. Carlsson J, Miketic S, Windeler J, et al. Randomized trial of rate-control vs. rhythm-control in persistent atrial fibrillation: the Strategies of Treatment of Atrial Fibrillation (STAF) study. *J Am Coll Cardiol.* 2003;41(10):1690–96.

5. Opolski G, Torbicki A, Kosior DA, et al. Rate control vs rhythm control in patients with nonvalvular persistent atrial fibrillation: the results of the Polish How to Treat Chronic Atrial Fibrillation (HOT CAFE) Study. *Chest.* 2004;126(2):476–86.

6. Roy D, Talajic M, Nattel S, et al. Rhythm control vs. rate control for atrial fibrillation and heart failure. *N Engl J Med.* 2008;358(25):2667–77.

7. Kober L, Torp-Pedersen C, McMurray JJ, et al. Increased mortality after dronedarone therapy for severe heart failure. *N Engl J Med.* 2008;358(25):2678–87.

8. Ionescu-Ittu R, Abrahamowicz M, Jackeviscius CA, et al. Comparative effectiveness of rhythm control vs rate control drug treatment effect on mortality in patients with atrial fibrillation. *Arch Intern Med.* 2012;172(13):997.

9. Dewland TA, Marcus GM. Rate vs rhythm control in atrial fibrillation: can observational data trump randomized trial results? *Arch Intern Med.* 2012;172(13):983.

11

Early Use of the Pulmonary Artery Catheter and Outcomes in Patients with Shock and Acute Respiratory Distress Syndrome

A Randomized Controlled Trial

[C]linical management involving early use of a [pulmonary artery catheter] was not associated with significant changes in mortality and morbidity among patients with shock, [acute respiratory distress syndrome], or both.

—RICHARD ET AL.[1]

Research Question: Do critically ill patients benefit from early insertion of a pulmonary artery catheter to help guide management?[1]

Funding: Two French governmental agencies and a company that manufactures medical devices.

Year Study Began: 1999.

Year Study Published: 2003.

Study Location: 36 intensive care units in France.

Who Was Studied: Patients with shock, acute respiratory distress syndrome (ARDS), or both.

Who Was Excluded: Patients with hemorrhagic shock, those with a myocardial infarction complicated by cardiogenic shock and requiring revascularization, and those with a platelet count ≤10,000 per microliter. In addition, patients meeting criteria for shock for longer than 12 hours were excluded.

How Many Patients: 676.

Study Overview: See Figure 11.1 for an overview of the study's design.

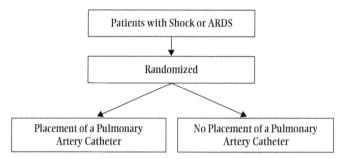

Figure 11.1 Summary of the trial design.

Study Intervention: Patients assigned to the pulmonary artery catheter group received a catheter within 2 hours of enrollment. The type of catheter was determined by the care team, as was the site of catheter insertion. Additionally, the decision about when to remove the catheter or whether to replace it was left to the care team. The care team could use data from the catheter to guide therapy (e.g., physicians could adjust medications based on the pressure readings), but the care team was not given specific protocols to follow.

Patients in the control group did not receive a catheter but otherwise received standard care.

Follow-Up: 28 days.

Endpoints: Primary outcome: mortality after 28 days. Secondary outcomes: length of stay in the hospital and intensive care unit (ICU), organ system failure, and the need for mechanical ventilation, dialysis, or vasoactive medications.

RESULTS

- In the control group, a pulmonary artery catheter was inserted in 4.4% of patients despite the fact that this violated the study protocol.

- In the catheter group, 2.4% of patients did not receive a catheter (six died before catheter insertion, whereas in two patients, catheter placement was not possible).
- In patients in the catheter group, the catheter remained in place for a mean of 2.3 days.
- During catheter insertion, approximately 5% of patients experienced an arterial puncture and approximately 18% experienced arrhythmias or conduction disturbances; there were no deaths directly attributable to catheter insertion, however.
- There were no significant differences in mortality between patients in the pulmonary artery catheter group and control group (Table 11.1).
- There were also no significant differences between patients in the pulmonary artery catheter group and patients in the control group with respect to organ system failure or the need for mechanical ventilation, dialysis, or vasoactive medications.

Table 11.1. SUMMARY OF THE TRIAL'S KEY FINDINGS

Outcome	Pulmonary Artery Catheter Group	Control Group	P Value
28-day mortality	59.4%	61%	0.67
Intensive care unit length of stay	11.6 days	11.9 days	0.72
Hospital length of stay	14 days	14.4 days	0.67

Criticisms and Limitations: The study was underpowered for detecting small differences in outcomes between patients in the catheter vs. control groups.

Physicians treating patients in the catheter group used data from the pulmonary artery catheters to guide therapy, but they were not given specific protocols to follow. It is possible that catheterization might have resulted in a significant benefit if the care teams had been given management protocols.

Other Relevant Studies and Information:

- A number of other randomized trials in critically ill patients have also failed to show a benefit of pulmonary artery catheterization.[2,3]
- A trial of pulmonary artery catheterization in patients admitted to the hospital for heart failure did not demonstrate a benefit,[4] nor did a trial of pulmonary artery catheterization in high-risk patients before surgery.[5]

- Because of these findings, pulmonary artery catheters are used much less commonly now than in the past.[6]

Summary and Implications: In critically ill patients, pulmonary artery catheterization did not lead to improved outcomes compared with standard care without catheterization. This trial, along with other trials of pulmonary artery catheterization, demonstrates the importance of evaluating widely used technologies that have never been adequately assessed.

CLINICAL CASE: PULMONARY ARTERY CATHETERS IN CRITICALLY ILL PATIENTS

Case History

A 60-year-old man was admitted to the intensive care unit 36 hours ago with severe pancreatitis. He was intubated on admission because of tachypnea and hypoxemia. He continues to have a high oxygen requirement with a Pao_2 of 95 mm Hg despite receiving an Fio_2 of 0.60. His chest radiograph shows bilateral pulmonary infiltrates, and an echocardiogram shows no evidence of cardiac dysfunction.

The attending pulmonologist would like to place a pulmonary artery catheter to help guide management. She says, "How else am I supposed to know whether the patient needs more diuresis?"

Based on the results of this trial of pulmonary artery catheterization, do you agree with the pulmonologist's recommendation?

Suggested Answer

Existing data, including this trial, do not suggest that pulmonary artery catheterization in critically ill patients is beneficial. In addition, pulmonary artery catheterization may lead to complications (according to this trial, the risk for arterial puncture is approximately 5%, whereas the risk for arrhythmias or conduction disturbances is approximately 18%). Therefore, pulmonary artery catheterization is generally not indicated for patients like the one in this vignette. This patient's volume status should be monitored using clinical findings and other data.

References

1. Richard C, Warsawski J, Anguel N, et al. Early use of the pulmonary artery catheter and outcomes in patients with shock and acute respiratory distress syndrome. *JAMA*. 2003;290(20): 2713–20.
2. Shah MR, Hasselblad V, Stevenson LW, et al. Impact of the pulmonary artery catheter in critically ill patients: meta-analysis of randomized clinical trials. *JAMA*. 2005;294(13):1664.
3. National Heart, Lung, and Blood Institute Acute Respiratory Distress Syndrome (ARDS) Clinical Trials Network. Pulmonary-artery vs. central venous catheter to guide treatment of acute lung injury. *N Engl J Med*. 2006;354(21):2213.
4. Binanay C, Califf RM, Hasselblad V, et al. Evaluation study of congestive heart failure and pulmonary artery catheterization effectiveness: the ESCAPE trial. *JAMA*. 2005;294(13):1625.
5. Sandham JD, Hull RD, Brant RF, et al. A randomized, controlled trial of the use of pulmonary-artery catheters in high-risk surgical patients. *N Engl J Med*. 2003;348(1):5.
6. Koo KK, Sun JC, Zhou Q, et al. Pulmonary artery catheters: evolving rates and reasons for use. *Crit Care Med*. 2011;39(7):1613.

12

Statins and Perioperative Cardiac Complications

> Use of statins was highly protective against perioperative cardiac complications in patients undergoing vascular surgery in this retrospective study.
>
> —O'NEIL-CALLAHAN ET AL.[1]

Research Question: Do statins decrease perioperative cardiac complications in patients undergoing noncardiac vascular surgery?

Year Study Published: 2005.

Study Location: Beth Israel Deaconess Medical Center, Boston, Massachusetts.

Who Was Studied: All patients who underwent carotid endarterectomy, aortic surgery (aortoiliac bypass, aneurysm, or dissection repair), or peripheral lower extremity revascularization not involving the aorta between January 1999 and December 2000.

How Many Patients: 997.

Study Overview: See Figure 12.1 for an overview of the study's design.

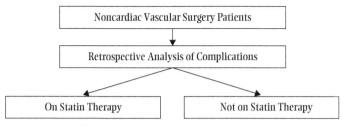

Figure 12.1 Summary of the study design.

Study Intervention: In this retrospective study, medical records were retrieved and standardized forms used to extract data on patient characteristics, perioperative care, and complications occurring during the index hospitalization. Data were analyzed to determine whether statin use was associated with a decreased risk for perioperative cardiac complications and if findings were independent of other contributing factors.

Follow-Up: From day of surgery until day of discharge.

Endpoints: Primary outcome: occurrence of complications (death, acute myocardial infarction [MI], myocardial ischemia, acute congestive heart failure, ventricular tachyarrhythmias). Secondary outcome: time of onset of complications (days after surgery).

RESULTS

- A total of 1,163 hospitalizations were analyzed for 997 patients. The study population was predominantly older adult men with a high prevalence of smoking, diabetes, hypertension, and cardiac disease. In approximately half of the cases, statins, beta blockers, aspirin, and angiotensin-converting enzyme (ACE) inhibitors were given.
- Complications of interest were found in 157 hospitalizations: 52 (9.9%) of 526 hospitalizations in the statin group vs. 105 (16.5%) of 637 hospitalizations in the group not taking statins (number needed to treat = 15) (Table 12.1).
- There was no difference in the timing of complications between the two groups.
- For all complications, the odds ratio (OR) was 0.56 (95% confidence interval 0.39 to 0.79, P = 0.0012). The OR was 0.56 and statistically significant for the combined endpoints of death, MI, and myocardial

ischemia (driven by myocardial ischemia without a clearly demonstrated benefit for deaths or MIs).

- On multivariate analysis accounting for age, gender, body mass index (BMI), surgery type and acuity, left ventricular dysfunction, and diabetes, statin use was associated with a significant reduction in rate of complications. Subgroup analysis showed no statistically significant differences between any subgroups of interest.
- Aside from statins, no other pharmacologic intervention was retained as an independent predictor of the complication rate. When beta blockers were considered in the multivariate model, the protective effect of statins remained unchanged, whereas beta blockers had no clear effect.
- Statin use was associated with hypercholesterolemia, carotid surgery, beta blockers, and higher BMI and was inversely associated with nonelective surgery or other antilipidemic therapy. The benefits of statins remained unchanged after adjusting for the derived propensity score.

Table 12.1. SUMMARY OF KEY FINDINGS*

Complication Outcomes	RECEIVING STATINS Hospitalizations = 526 Total Complications = 52 % (*N*)	NOT RECEIVING STATINS Hospitalizations = 637 Total Complications = 105 % (*N*)
Death	1.1 (6)	0.78 (5)
Myocardial infarction	1.3 (7)	1.1 (7)
Other ischemia	1 (5)	4.1 (26)
Congestive heart failure	4 (21)	7.8 (50)
Ventricular tachyarrhythmia	2.5 (13)	2.7 (17)

*For patients with more than one of the complications, only the outcome higher on the list was counted.

Criticisms and Limitations: Since this was a retrospective and nonrandomized study, the results may have been affected by unmeasured confounding factors.

Other Relevant Studies and Information:

- A meta-analysis of randomized controlled trials examined whether preprocedural statin therapy reduced periprocedural cardiovascular events following invasive procedures. A total of 21 trials and 4,805 patients were included in the analysis. The use of statins before invasive procedures significantly reduced the hazard of postprocedural MI and the risk for atrial fibrillation after coronary artery bypass grafting.[2]

- A meta-analysis of randomized controlled trials examined whether short-term statin therapy (commenced before or on the day of elective, noncardiac vascular surgery and continued for at least 48 hours afterward) had an effect on patient outcomes (risk for complications, pain, quality of life, and length of hospital stay) at different dosages. Evidence was insufficient to allow for a conclusion of whether short-term perioperative statin use had an effect on any of the outcomes examined.[3]

- The 2014 guidelines from the American College/American Heart Association (ACC/AHA)[4] on perioperative management for noncardiac surgery indicate that "statins should be continued in patients currently taking statins and scheduled for noncardiac surgery." (Box 12.1).

BOX 12.1. 2014 ACC/AHA GUIDELINES FOR PERIOPERATIVE STATIN THERAPY

Class I Recommendation
Statins should be continued in patients currently taking statins and scheduled for noncardiac surgery.
(Level of Evidence: B)

Class IIa Recommendation
Perioperative initiation of statin use is reasonable in patients undergoing vascular surgery.
(Level of Evidence: B)

Class IIb Recommendation
Perioperative initiation of statins may be considered in patients with clinical indications according to guideline-directed medical therapy who are undergoing elevated-risk procedures.
(Level of Evidence: C)

Summary and Implications: This retrospective study suggests a protective effect of statins with respect to perioperative cardiac complications in patients undergoing vascular surgery. The accumulated evidence to date suggests a protective

effect of perioperative statin use on cardiac complications during noncardiac surgery, but randomized controlled trials are needed to confirm this finding. Current
guidelines indicate that "statins should be continued in patients currently taking
statins and scheduled for noncardiac surgery."

CLINICAL CASE: PERIOPERATIVE STATIN THERAPY

Case History
A 55-year-old man presents to the preoperative clinic for evaluation before undergoing a vascular surgery procedure. The patient has brought his
list of home medications (which includes a statin agent) and asks which
medications he should continue taking. What is the recommendation regarding perioperative statin therapy?

Suggested Answer
According to the ACC/AHA guidelines, statins should be continued
perioperatively in this patient.

References

1. O'Neil-Callahan K, Katsimaglis G, Tepper MR, et al. Statins decrease perioperative
   cardiac complications in patients undergoing noncardiac vascular surgery: the
   Statins for Risk Reduction in Surgery (StaRRS) study. *J Am Coll Cardiol*. 2005 Feb
   1;45(3):336–42.
2. Winchester DE, Wen X, Xie L, Bavry AA. Evidence of pre-procedural statin
   therapy: a meta-analysis of randomized trials. *J AM Coll Cardiol*. 2010 Sep
   28;56(14):1099–109.
3. Sanders RD, Nicholson A, Lewis SR, Smith AF, Alderson P. Perioperative statin
   therapy for improving outcomes during and after noncardiac vascular surgery.
   Cochrane Database Syst Rev. 2013 Jul 3;7:CD009971.
4. Fleisher LA, Fleischmann KE, Auerbach AD, et al. 2014 ACC/AHA guideline on perioperative cardiovascular evaluation and management of patient
   undergoing noncardiac surgery: a report of the American College/American
   Heart Association Task Force on Practice Guidelines. *Circulation*. 2014 Dec
   9;130(24):e278–333.

13

A Survey of Transesophageal Echocardiography

> This multicenter survey documents that TEE studies are associated with an acceptable low risk when used by experienced operators under proper safety conditions.
>
> —Daniel et al.[1]

Research Question: Is transesophageal echocardiography (TEE) a practical and safe technique?

Year Study Began: 1988.

Year Study Published: 1991.

Study Location: 15 centers in European countries (Germany, Italy, the Netherlands).

Who Was Studied: Centers performing TEE studies in adults for at least 1 year with detailed records of patients, side effects, and complications related to TEE.

How Many Patients: 10,419.

Study Overview: See Figure 13.1 for an overview of the study's design.

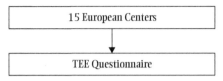

Figure 13.1 Summary of the study design.

Study Intervention: Data was collected with a detailed questionnaire regarding TEE examinations.

Endpoints: Survey questions covered a range of topics, including frequency of TEE procedures, training of operators, patient premedication, contraindications, and complications.

RESULTS

- At the time of the survey, 10,419 TEE examinations had been performed, ranging from 106 to 2,977 studies per center. All centers performed transthoracic echocardiography (TTE) before TEE. All centers used a one-lead electrocardiogram for continuous monitoring during TEE. Sedation was not used routinely. Local pharyngeal anesthesia was administered in all except one center. The majority of centers performed the exam in the left lateral decubitus position.
- Patients ranged from 9 to 84 years old. Of the 10,419 patients, 9,240 (88.7%) were conscious during their TEE exam (inpatient or outpatient), with minimum fasting times ranging between 3 to 9 hours. The remaining 1,179 patients underwent a TEE in the operating room or during mechanical ventilation in the intensive care unit.
- TEE was performed by physicians, 54% of whom had prior endoscopy training.
- In 201 of the TEE examinations (1.9%), the insertion of the probe was unsuccessful, and 198 of these failures (98.5%) were due to lack of patient cooperation and/or operator experience. The remaining failures were due to anatomic reasons (tracheostomy, esophageal diverticulum). Centers that performed fewer TEE examinations had higher rates of unsuccessful probe placement; in the four centers that had performed 200 or fewer TEE examinations, the failure of probe insertion averaged 3.9% ± 3.2% vs. 1.4% ± 0.9% in institutions that had performed more than 200 TEE examinations ($P < 0.05$).

- Ninety of the 10,218 TEE examinations with successful probe insertion (0.88%) were interrupted before completion because of intolerance of TEE probe (65 patients), serious cardiopulmonary or bleeding complications (18 patients, 0.18%), or other causes (vomiting, probe defect). In one patient, TEE resulted in severe hematemesis, ultimately leading to death (mortality rate of 0.0098%); on autopsy, a lung tumor was found to be penetrating the esophagus.

Criticisms and Limitations: Centers were included in the survey if detailed records of TEE examinations were available; this retrospective study cannot guarantee uniformity in data collection and adverse event reporting across study centers.

Other Relevant Studies and Information:

- A single-center series of 7,200 adult cardiac surgical patients[2] reported the incidences of TEE-associated morbidity and mortality in the study population to be 0.2% and 0%, respectively. TEE-associated complications: severe odynophagia (0.1%), dental injury (0.03%), endotracheal tube malpositioning (0.03%), upper gastrointestinal hemorrhage (0.03%), and esophageal perforation (0.01%). TEE probe insertion was unsuccessful or contraindicated in 0.18% and 0.5% of the study population, respectively.
- A systematic review[3] of 13 studies was conducted examining the perioperative use of point-of-care TTE/TEE in noncardiac surgery for high-risk patients or during periods of hemodynamic compromise/ cardiac arrest. The most frequent diagnoses were valvulopathies, low ejection fraction, hypovolemia, pulmonary embolism, severe wall motion abnormalities, and right ventricular failure.

Summary and Implications: This multicenter survey found the complication rate associated with TEE to be low; however, serious complications did occur, necessitating a risk-benefit analysis before the procedure. Centers that performed fewer TEE examinations had higher probe insertion failure rates, indicating the presence of a learning curve. TEE should be performed by experienced physicians in facilities that allow prompt cardiopulmonary resuscitation.

CLINICAL CASE: INTRAOPERATIVE TEE

Case History

A 77-year-old man presents for aortic valve replacement and two-vessel CABG at a center that routinely performs intraoperative TEE during cardiac surgery. During the preoperative evaluation, it is explained to the patient that an intraoperative TEE will be performed. The patient expresses concern about possible complications associated with the TEE procedure. How should the patient's concerns be addressed?

Suggested Answer

Possible complications of TEE, such as odynophagia, dental injury, or esophageal injury, should be discussed. The patient should be reassured that the overall incidence of TEE-associated morbidity is low (on the order of 0.2%).

References

1. Daniel WG, Erbel R, Kasper W, et al. Safety of transesophageal echocardiography: a multicenter survey of 10,419 examinations. *Circulation.* 1991 Mar;83(3):817–21.
2. Kallmeyer IJ, Collard CD, Fox JA, Body SC, Shernan SK. The safety of intraoperative transesophageal echocardiography: a case series of 7200 cardiac surgical patients. *Anesth Analg.* 2001 May;92(5):1126–30.
3. Jasudavisius A, Arellano R, Martin J, McConnell B, Bainbridge D. A systematic review of transthoracic and transesophageal echocardiography in non-cardiac surgery: implications for point-of-care ultrasound education in the operating room. *Can J Anaesth.* 2016 Apr;63(4):480–87.

14

Statins and Perioperative Cardiac Complications

[Patients with three-vessel and/or left main coronary artery disease] treated with [percutaneous coronary intervention] involving drug-eluting stents were more likely than those undergoing [coronary artery bypass grafting] to reach the primary end point of the study—death from any cause, stroke, myocardial infarction, or repeat revascularization. . . . [However, patients undergoing stenting] were less likely to have a stroke.

—LANGE AND HILLIS[1]

Research Question: Should patients with severe coronary artery disease (three-vessel and/or left main disease) be treated with percutaneous coronary intervention (PCI) or coronary artery bypass grafting (CABG)?[2]

Funding: Boston Scientific, which manufactures cardiac stents.

Year Study Began: 2005.

Year Study Published: 2009.

Study Location: 85 sites in 17 countries in the United States and Europe.

Who Was Studied: Patients with ≥50% stenosis in at least three coronary arteries or in the left main coronary artery in whom "equivalent anatomical revascularization could be achieved with either CABG or PCI" as judged by a cardiologist and cardiac surgeon. Patients were also required to have symptoms of stable or unstable angina, atypical chest pain, or, if asymptomatic, evidence of myocardial ischemia on a stress test.

Who Was Excluded: Patients with prior PCI or CABG, those with an acute myocardial infarction (MI), and those requiring another cardiac surgery.

How Many Patients: 1,800.

Study Overview: See Figure 14.1 for an overview of the study's design.

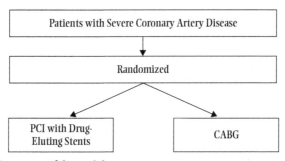

Figure 14.1 Summary of the trial design.

Study Intervention: Patients assigned to both the PCI and CABG groups underwent the procedures according to local practice. Patients in the PCI group received drug-eluting stents. The goal of therapy in both groups was complete revascularization of all target vessels. Adjunctive periprocedural and postprocedural therapy, including antiplatelet therapy, was also provided according to local practice.

Follow-Up: 12 months.

Endpoints: Primary outcome: a composite of major cardiovascular and cerebrovascular events (death from any cause, stroke, MI, or repeat revascularization). Each component of this composite was also assessed individually.

RESULTS

- The mean age of study participants was 65 years; approximately 25% had diabetes, 57% had stable angina, 28% had unstable angina, and 2% had an ejection fraction <30%.

- Patients in the PCI group received an average of more than four stents each.
- Patients in the PCI group had a shorter length of hospital stay (3.4 days vs. 9.5 days, $P < 0.001$).
- Patients in the PCI group received more aggressive postprocedure medication therapy (e.g., more patients received antiplatelet medications, warfarin, statins, and angiotensin-converting enzyme inhibitors); however, more patients in the CABG group received amiodarone.
- Patients in the CABG group had lower rates of total cardiovascular and cerebrovascular events than those in the PCI group but a higher rate of stroke (Table 14.1).
- The authors also report stratified patient outcomes using a prediction rule—called the SYNTAX score—that classifies coronary artery disease by its complexity (e.g., lesions that are anatomically more difficult to access with PCI receive a higher score); patients with higher SYNTAX scores, that is, more complex lesions, appear to benefit more from CABG vs. PCI than do patients with lower SYNTAX scores; the SYNTAX score may be helpful in identifying which patients are most likely to benefit from CABG.

Table 14.1. SUMMARY OF SYNTAX's KEY FINDINGS

Outcome	PCI Group	CABG Group	P Value
Major cardiovascular or cerebrovascular events	17.8%	12.4%	0.002
Death	4.4%	3.5%	0.37
Stroke	0.6%	2.2%	0.003
Myocardial infarction	4.8%	3.3%	0.11
Repeat revascularization	13.5%	5.9%	<0.001
Freedom from angina[3]	71.6%	76.3%	0.05

Criticisms and Limitations: If patients in the CABG group had received postprocedure medication therapy similar to that received by patients in the PCI group, the benefits of CABG vs. PCI may have been more pronounced.

In addition, the study only involved 22% female patients and thus may not be applicable to female patients.

Finally, patients in the PCI group were given paclitaxel-eluting TAXUS stents, which are believed to be less effective than some other brands of drug-eluting stents.

Other Relevant Studies and Information:

- A 3-year follow up analysis was consistent with the 12-month findings: major cardiovascular or cerebrovascular events remained significantly higher in the PCI vs. CABG group (28% vs. 20.2%), and most of the difference was attributable primarily to higher rates of repeat revascularization with PCI.[4]
- Trials before the advent of drug-eluting stents that compared PCI with CABG in patients with multivessel disease demonstrated results similar to SYNTAX.[5]
- An observational study suggested a long-term survival benefit of CABG vs. PCI among patients with multivessel coronary disease.[6]
- The STICH trial, which compared coronary-artery bypass surgery with medical therapy in patients with coronary artery disease and an ejection fraction ≤35%, found that the two treatments led to similar mortality rates.[7]

Summary and Implications: For patients with three-vessel and/or left main coronary artery disease, CABG reduced rates of major cardiovascular and cerebrovascular events compared with PCI. This difference was largely driven by a reduction in the need for repeat revascularization procedures among patients receiving CABG. Patients who received PCI had a lower rate of stroke, however, which may make PCI an attractive option for some patients. In addition, the authors suggest that patients with less complex coronary artery disease (as assessed using the SYNTAX score) may be particularly good candidates for PCI, but this hypothesis requires further validation.

CLINICAL CASE: CARDIAC STENTS VS. CORONARY ARTERY BYPASS SURGERY AMONG PATIENTS WITH SEVERE CORONARY ARTERY DISEASE

Case History

An 86-year-old man visits his doctor because of increasing shortness of breath when walking. The symptoms have been getting progressively worse over the past month. At baseline, the patient could walk for three blocks without resting, and now he can barely walk for one block. A cardiac stress test with nuclear imaging demonstrates reversible ischemia in the territory of the left main coronary artery.

Based on the results of the SYNTAX trial, do you believe that this patient should be treated with PCI or with CABG?

Suggested Answer

SYNTAX showed that, for patients with three-vessel and/or left main coronary artery disease, CABG lowered rates of major cardiovascular and cerebrovascular events compared with PCI. However, patients in the CABG group experienced a higher rate of stroke.

The patient in this vignette is much older than the typical patient in SYNTAX (approximately 65 years). Because of his advanced age and limited performance status, the less invasive treatment—PCI—would likely be preferable for him. In addition, he would be less likely to experience a stroke—which could be a devastating complication for him at this stage in his life. This case highlights why, despite the fact that CABG proved superior to PCI in SYNTAX, some patients may still reasonably opt for PCI.

References

1. Lange RA, Hillis LD. Coronary revascularization in context. *N Engl J Med.* 2009;360:1024–26.
2. Serruys PW, Morice MC, Kappetein AP, et al. Percutaneous coronary intervention vs. coronary-artery bypass grafting for severe coronary artery disease. *N Engl J Med.* 2009;360(10):961–72.
3. Cohen DJ, Van Hout B, Serruys PW, et al. Quality of life after PCI with drug-eluting stents or coronary artery bypass surgery. *N Engl J Med.* 2011;364:1016–26.
4. Kappetein AP, Feldman TE, Mack MJ, et al. Comparison of coronary bypass surgery with drug-eluting stenting for the treatment of left main and/or three-vessel disease: 3-year follow-up of the SYNTAX trial. *Eur Heart J.* 2011;32(17):2125–34.
5. Daemen J, Boersma E, Flather M, et al. Long-term safety and efficacy of percutaneous coronary intervention with stenting and coronary artery bypass surgery for multivessel coronary artery disease: a meta-analysis with 5-year patient-level data from the ARTS, ERACI-II, MASS-II, and SoS trials. *Circulation* 2008;118:1146–54.
6. Weintraub WS, Grau-Sepulveda MV, Weiss JM, et al. Comparative effectiveness of revascularization strategies. *N Engl J Med.* 2012;366(16):1467.
7. Velazquez EJ, Lee KL, Deja MA, et al. Coronary-artery bypass surgery in patients with left ventricular dysfunction. *N Engl J Med.* 2011;364:1607–16.

Effects of Extended-Release Metoprolol Succinate in Patients Undergoing Noncardiac Surgery (POISE Trial)

A Randomized Controlled Trial

[Although perioperative metoprolol] reduced the risk of myocardial infarction . . . compared with placebo, the drug also resulted in a significant excess risk of death, stroke, and clinically significant hypotension and bradycardia.

—POISE Study Group[1]

Research Question: Should patients undergoing noncardiac surgery receive a perioperative beta blocker to prevent cardiovascular complications?[1]

Funding: Governmental agencies from Canada, Australia, Spain, and Great Britain. AstraZeneca also provided a small portion of the funding.

Year Study Began: 2002.

Year Study Published: 2008.

Who Was Studied: Adults ≥45 years undergoing noncardiac surgery with an expected hospital length of stay ≥24 hours who had or were at risk for atherosclerotic disease. Patients undergoing elective, urgent, and emergent surgeries were all included.

Who Was Excluded: Patients with a heart rate <50 beats per minute, those with a second- or third-degree heart block, and those with asthma (because beta blockers can trigger asthma exacerbations). In addition, patients were excluded if they were already receiving a beta blocker or verapamil, had a known history of an adverse reaction to beta blockers, or were undergoing a "low-risk surgical procedure (based on the individual physician's judgment)."

How Many Patients: 8,351.

Study Overview: See Figure 15.1 for an overview of the study's design.

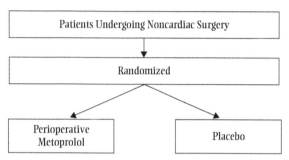

Figure 15.1 Summary of the POISE study design.

Study Intervention: Patients assigned to the metoprolol group received oral extended-release metoprolol starting 2–4 hours before surgery. Patients had their blood pressure and heart rate measured before medication administration, and the dose was held in patients with a heart rate <50 beats per minute or a systolic blood pressure <100 mm Hg. Patients also received postoperative extended-release metoprolol as follows:

- At any point in the first 6 hours following surgery, patients received a dose of metoprolol 100 mg if the heart rate was ≥80 beats per minute and the systolic blood pressure ≥100 mm Hg.
- Patients who did not receive metoprolol within the first 6 hours received a 100-mg dose 6 hours after surgery.
- Twelve hours after the first postoperative dose, patients began taking metoprolol 200 mg daily for 30 days.
- Metoprolol was held and the dose was reduced to 100 mg once daily in patients who had a heart rate <50 beats per minut4e or a systolic blood pressure <100 mm Hg.

Patients who could not take oral medications received intravenous metoprolol until they were able to tolerate oral medications.

Patients assigned to the placebo group were treated with placebo according to the same schedule.

Follow-Up: 30 days.

Endpoints: Primary outcome: a composite of cardiovascular death, non-fatal myocardial infarction, and nonfatal cardiac arrest at 30 days. Secondary outcomes: clinically significant hypotension, clinically significant bradycardia, stroke, and death.

RESULTS

- Data from 752 patients were excluded because of fraudulent activity, and data from 8,351 patients were analyzed in the final analysis.
- The mean age of study subjects was 69 years, the mean preoperative heart rate was 78 beats per minute, and the mean preoperative blood pressure was 139/78 mm Hg.
- Forty-two percent of patients underwent vascular surgery, 22% intraperitoneal surgery, and 21% orthopedic surgery.
- Patients in the metoprolol group had fewer myocardial infarctions than those in the control group but a higher rate of stroke and death (Table 15.1).

Table 15.1. SUMMARY OF POISE's KEY FINDINGS

Outcome	Metoprolol Group	Placebo Group	P Value
Cardiovascular death, myocardial infarction, and cardiac arrest	5.8%	6.9%	0.039
Nonfatal myocardial infarction*	3.6%	5.1%	0.0008
Clinically significant hypotension	15.0%	9.7%	<0.0001
Clinically significant bradycardia	6.6%	2.4%	<0.0001
Stroke	1.0%	0.5%	0.0053
Death	3.1%	2.3%	0.0317

*Two-thirds of the myocardial infarctions did not result in ischemic symptoms. Myocardial infarctions in these patients were diagnosed based on elevations of cardiac biomarkers and an additional defining feature of myocardial infarction (e.g., ischemic electrocardiogram changes or wall motion abnormalities on an echocardiogram).

Criticisms and Limitations: It is possible that the results would have been different if a different beta blocker or different dose had been used or if the medication had been given according to a different dosing schedule.

Other Relevant Studies and Information:

- A meta-analysis of more than 30 trials evaluating the use of perioperative beta blockers was consistent with POISE.[2]
- Small trials using low-dose beta blockers[3] and in which the beta blocker was initiated at least 1 week before surgery[4] have suggested a benefit of perioperative beta blockade in preventing cardiovascular complications; however, there were methodologic limitations to these studies, and the reliability of the results of one of these studies has been called into question.[4]
- Guidelines published after POISE emphasize that evidence supporting initiation of perioperative beta blockade is weak. When beta blockers are initiated perioperatively—something that is not necessarily recommended—they should only be given to high-risk patients undergoing intermediate- to high-risk surgeries and should be started at low doses (target heart rate 60–80 beats per minute) at least a week beforehand. Patients already receiving beta blockers should be continued on them perioperatively, however, because rapid withdrawal of beta blockers may lead to cardiovascular complications.[5]

Summary and Implications: The initiation of perioperative extended-release metoprolol in patients not currently taking a beta blocker lowers the risk for myocardial infarction but leads to clinically significant bradycardia and hypotension and increases the risk for stroke and overall mortality. It is possible that, when initiated at least several days before surgery and at appropriate doses, perioperative beta blockers may benefit some high-risk patients. However, existing evidence does not provide support for the initiation of perioperative beta blockers in most patients not currently taking these medications.

CLINICAL CASE: PERIOPERATIVE BETA BLOCKADE

Case History

A 70-year-old woman is brought to the emergency department by ambulance after a bystander found her clutching her abdomen on the street. The patient is in severe pain and tells you she has "heart problems" but cannot recall her medications. Her heart rate is 110 beats per minute, and her blood pressure is 160/100 mm Hg. A computed tomography scan of her abdomen shows evidence of an acute intra-abdominal process, and she is scheduled for an urgent laparotomy.

Based on the results of POISE, should you treat this patient with a perioperative beta blocker?

Suggested Answer

The POISE trial does not support the routine initiation of perioperative beta blockers in patients undergoing noncardiac surgery. However, patients chronically receiving beta blockers were excluded from POISE because rapid withdrawal of beta blockers may lead to cardiovascular complications.

We do not know whether the patient in this vignette regularly receives a beta blocker. If she does, the beta blocker should be continued as long as her heart rate and blood pressure can tolerate it. But if she doesn't, a beta blocker probably should not be started.

Given the uncertainty, common sense should be used in managing this patient. Because she has cardiovascular disease and her heart rate and blood pressure are elevated, it might be reasonable to cautiously initiate a low-dose, short-acting beta blocker and monitor her carefully for bradycardia and hypotension. However, it would be equally correct to withhold a beta blocker, particularly postoperatively because monitoring on surgical floors is often sparse.

References

1. POISE Study Group. Effects of extended-release metoprolol succinate in patients undergoing non-cardiac surgery (POISE trial): a randomised controlled trial. *Lancet.* 2008;371(9627):1839–47.
2. Bangalore S, Wetterslev J, Pranesh S, et al. Perioperative beta blockers in patients having non-cardiac surgery: a meta-analysis. *Lancet.* 2008;372(9654):1962.
3. Mangano DT, Layug EL, Wallace A, Tateo I. Effect of atenolol on mortality and cardiovascular morbidity after noncardiac surgery. *N Engl J Med.* 1996;335:1713–20.
4. Poldermans D, Boersma E, Bax JJ, et al. The effect of bisoprolol on perioperative mortality and myocardial infarction in high-risk patients undergoing vascular surgery. *N Engl J Med.* 1999;341:1789–94.
5. American College of Cardiology Foundation/American Heart Association Task Force on Practice Guidelines. 2009 ACCF/AHA focused update on perioperative beta blockade. *J Am Coll Cardiol.* 2009;54(22):2102.

SECTION 3

Neuroanesthesia

16

Adverse Cerebral Outcomes After Coronary Bypass Surgery

Adverse cerebral outcomes after coronary bypass surgery are relatively common and serious; they are associated with substantial increases in mortality, length of hospitalization, and use of intermediate- or long-term care facilities.

—ROACH ET AL.[1]

Research Question: For patients undergoing elective coronary bypass surgery, what are the incidence and predictors of perioperative adverse neurologic events, and what is the impact of neurologic outcomes on resource utilization?

Funding: Ischemia Research and Education Foundation.

Year Study Began: 1991.

Year Study Published: 1996.

Study Location: 24 institutions in the United States.

Who Was Studied: Adult patients undergoing elective coronary artery bypass grafting (CABG) surgery over a 2-year period.

Who Was Excluded: Patients who could not be evaluated for neurologic outcomes, had undergone concomitant intracardiac or vascular procedures, or had died during surgery.

How Many Patients: 2,108.

Study Overview: See Figure 16.1 for an overview of the study's design.

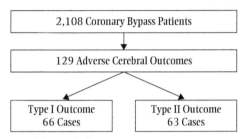

Figure 16.1 Summary of the study design.

Endpoints: New perioperative neurologic findings were classified into two categories: type I outcome (death due to stroke or hypoxic encephalopathy, nonfatal stroke, transient ischemic attack, or stupor or coma at the time of discharge) and type II outcome (new deterioration in intellectual function, confusion, agitation, disorientation, memory deficit, or seizure without evidence of focal injury). Resource utilization was evaluated by tracking the length of postoperative intensive care unit (ICU) and hospital stays as well as the discharge destination (home vs. intensive intermediate- or long-term care).

RESULTS

- Perioperative adverse cerebral outcomes occurred in 129 patients (6.1%). A type I neurologic outcome occurred in 66 cases (3.1%)—8 patients died of cerebral injury, 55 patients had nonfatal strokes, 2 patients had transient ischemic attacks, and 1 patient had stupor at the time of discharge. A type II neurologic outcome occurred in 63 cases (3%)—55 patients showed deterioration in intellectual function, and 8 patients had seizures.
- In-hospital mortality increased 10-fold for type I and 5-fold for type II outcomes. Average lengths of postsurgical ICU and hospital stays were doubled in patients with adverse cerebral outcomes (see Table 16.1 for summary of key findings).

- Patients with adverse cerebral outcomes had higher rates of discharge to facilities for intermediate- or long-term care: 47% of patients with type I and 30% of patients with type II outcomes were discharge to skilled nursing facilities or rehabilitation centers compared with 8% of patients without adverse cerebral outcomes.
- Predictors unique to type I outcomes were proximal aortic atherosclerosis, a history of neurologic disease, diabetes mellitus, and unstable angina. Predictors unique to type II outcomes were excessive alcohol consumption, prior CABG surgery, a history of peripheral vascular disease, and postoperative dysrhythmia.
- Predictors common to both type I and II neurologic outcomes were age (particularly ≥70 years), pulmonary disease, hypertension, and perioperative hypotension.

Table 16.1. SUMMARY OF KEY FINDINGS*

Variable	Type I Outcome (*N* = 66)	Type II Outcome (*N* = 63)	No Adverse Cerebral Event (*N* = 1979)
Death during hospitalization— no. (%)	14 (21)	6 (10)	38 (2)
Duration of postop hospital stay—days Median	17.6	10.9	7.7
Duration of ICU stay—days Median	5.8	3.2	1.9
Discharged to home— no. (%)[†]	21 (32)	38 (60)	1773 (90)

*P < 0.001 for all comparisons among the groups.
[†]Patients not discharged to home either died or were discharged to intermediate or long-term care facilities.

Criticisms and Limitations: Neurologic findings were not assessed by a single neurologist but by investigators at each participating study site. Neuropsychological deficits and deterioration in intellectual function were not independently evaluated because of resource constraints. Proximal aortic atherosclerosis was detected by palpation rather than more sensitive techniques, such as echocardiography. Carotid duplex scanning to detect carotid artery disease was not performed. The use of a left ventricular venting procedure and the occurrence of type I outcomes were weakly associated, but statistical assessment was limited by the small sample of patients without ventricular venting.

Other Relevant Studies and Information:

- In 2011, Misfeld et al.[2] published a metanalysis of eight observational studies comparing neurologic complications after off-pump CABG with and without aortic manipulation. Postsurgical neurologic complications were significantly lower in anaortic off-pump CABG cases (odds ratio = 0.46; 95% confidence interval = 0.29–0.72; P = 0.0008)

Summary and Implications: This prospective, multicenter investigation of adverse cerebral outcomes after elective CABG surgery found that 6.1% of patients experience adverse perioperative cerebral outcomes. The study also identified predictors of adverse cerebral outcomes and highlighted the significance and economic consequences of perioperative neurologic events.

CLINICAL CASE: RISK FOR PERIOPERATIVE NEUROLOGIC EVENTS

Case History

A 68-year-old patient is evaluated in the preoperative clinic before undergoing elective two-vessel CABG surgery. His past medical history is significant for hypertension and severe proximal aortic atherosclerosis. He is a practicing professor and concerned about intellectual function after the procedure. Based on the preoperative evaluation, how should this patient be managed to minimize the risk for adverse cerebral outcomes?

Suggested Answer

The risk for postoperative adverse cerebral outcomes needs to be discussed with the patient. Because of the presence of severe proximal aortic atherosclerosis and associated risk for adverse neurologic events, the surgical approach should aim to avoid manipulation of the proximal aorta if possible. Perioperative hypotension should be minimized.

References

1. Roach GW, Kanchuger K, Mangano CM, et al. Adverse cerebral outcomes after coronary bypass surgery. Multicenter Study of Perioperative Ischemia Research Group

and the Ischemia Research and Education Foundation Investigators. *N Engl J Med* 1996 Dec 19;335(25):1857–63.

2. Misfeld M, Brereton RJ, Sweetman EA, Doig GS. Neurologic complications after off-pump coronary artery bypass grafting with and without aortic manipulation: meta-analysis of 11,398 cases from 8 studies. *J Thorac Cardiovasc Surg.* 2011 Aug;142(2):e11–17.

17

Long-Term Cognitive Impairment After Critical Illness

A longer duration of delirium in the hospital was associated with worse global cognition and executive function scores at 3 and 12 months.
—PANDHARIPANDE ET AL.[1]

Research Question: What is the prevalence of long-term cognitive impairment after critical illness, and does the duration of delirium and use of sedative or analgesic medications affect cognitive outcomes?

Funding: National Institutes of Health, Veterans Affairs (VA) Clinical Science Research and Development Service, Foundation for Anesthesia Education and Research, VA Tennessee Valley Geriatric Research Education and Clinical Center.

Year Study Began: 2007.

Year Study Published: 2013.

Study Location: Vanderbilt University Medical Center and Saint Thomas Hospital in Nashville, Tennessee.

Who Was Studied: Adult patients with respiratory failure, cardiogenic shock, or septic shock admitted to a medical or surgical intensive care unit (ICU).

Who Was Excluded: Patients with substantial recent ICU exposure; those who could not be reliably assessed for delirium (blindness, deafness, inability to speak English); patients for whom follow-up would be difficult because of substance abuse, psychotic disorder, homelessness, or residence 200 miles or more from the enrolling center; patients unlikely to survive for 24 hours; patients for whom informed consent could not be obtained; those at high risk for preexisting cognitive deficits (neurodegenerative disease, recent cardiac surgery, suspected anoxic brain injury, or severe dementia); and patients with preexisting cognitive impairment (assessed using two validated scales).

How Many Patients: 821.

Study Overview: See Figure 17.1 for an overview of the study's design.

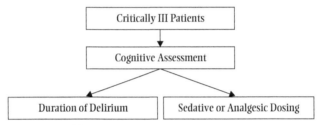

Figure 17.1 Summary of the study design.

Study Intervention: This multicenter, prospective cohort study involved a diverse population of critically ill ICU patients. Two validated measurement scales—the Confusion Assessment Method for the ICU (CAM-ICU)[2] and the Richmond Agitation-Sedation Scale (RASS)[3]—were used to assess baseline cognitive impairment as well as delirium and level of consciousness on a daily basis during hospitalization until hospital discharge or study day 30. Psychologists blinded to the hospital course administered tests to assess global cognition and executive function at 3 and 12 months after discharge using the Repeatable Battery for the Assessment of Neuropsychological Status (RBANS global cognition score)[4] and the Trail Making Test, Part B[5]. Medication-administration records were used to determine daily doses of benzodiazepines, opiates, propofol, and dexmedetomidine.

Follow-Up: 12 months.

Endpoints: Primary outcome: RBANS global cognition score at 3 and 12 months after discharge. Secondary outcomes: Trails B score and RBANS scores for immediate memory, delayed memory, and attention at 3 and 12 months after discharge.

RESULTS

- Patients in the study had a median age of 61 years and a high severity of illness. Only 6% of patients had cognitive impairment at baseline. Delirium affected 74% of patients during their hospital stay, with a median duration of 4 days.
- Between enrollment and the 3-month follow-up, 31% of patients died. Of the surviving patients, 79% underwent cognitive testing at 3 months after discharge. Another 7% of the original cohort died before the 12-month follow-up, and 75% of the surviving patients were tested at 12 months after discharge.
- Patients across all age groups and coexisting conditions had impaired global cognition scores at 3 and 12 months. Median RBANS global cognition scores at 3 and 12 months were approximately 1.5 SD below the age-adjusted population mean; such a decline was similar to scores for patients with mild cognitive impairment.
- At 3 months after discharge, 40% of patients had global cognition scores worse than those typically seen in patients with moderate traumatic brain injury, and 26% had scores 2 SD below the population means, which were similar to scores seen in patients with mild Alzheimer disease. At 12 months after discharge, the percentages were 34% and 24%, respectively.
- Trail B executive function scores were also low at 3 and 12 months after discharge.
- A longer duration of delirium was an independent risk factor for worse executive function and RBANS global cognition scores at 3 and 12 months after discharge.
- Higher benzodiazepine doses were an independent risk factor for worse executive function scores at 3 months ($P = 0.04$) but not at 12 months. None of the other medications examined were consistently associated with global cognition or executive function outcomes. After adjustment for delirium, there was no consistent association between sedative or analgesic medications and long-term cognitive impairment.

Criticisms and Limitations: Less than 50% of the original cohort of patients was included in the analysis at 12 months after discharge, leading to possible confounding due to death or withdrawal. The possibility of bias due to unmeasured confounding variables cannot be excluded. A formal evaluation of baseline cognitive function before illness was not possible.

Other Relevant Studies and Information:

- Several studies demonstrate that sedation confounds delirium assessment, especially when using the CAM-ICU, which determines the presence or absence of delirium based on four features: acute change or a fluctuation in mental status, inattention, disorganized thinking, and altered level of consciousness.[2,6]
- A prospective cohort study of 1,194 patients with 1,520 hospitalizations for severe sepsis examined the change in cognitive impairment and physical functioning after survival. Severe sepsis was independently associated with substantial and persistent new cognitive impairment and functional disability.[7]
- An observational study of 300 ICU patients examined the effects of a quality improvement project incorporating multifaceted sleep-promoting interventions. Significant improvements in perceived nighttime noise, incidence of delirium/coma, and daily delirium/coma-free status were demonstrated. Improvements in secondary outcomes (ICU and hospital length of stay and mortality) and post-ICU outcomes (cognition and perceived sleep quality) did not reach statistical significance.[8]

Summary and Implications: This study demonstrated that 74% of adult patients with critical illness experience delirium during their hospital course. Furthermore, patients in the ICU setting commonly experience global cognition and executive function deficits at 3 and 12 months following hospitalization. These findings highlight the importance of careful delirium surveillance in ICU patients.

References

1. Pandharipande PP, Girard TD, Jackson JC, et al. Long-term cognitive impairment after critical illness. *N Engl J Med.* 2013 Oct 3;369(14):1306–16.
2. Ely EW, Inouye SK, Bernard GR, et al. Delirium in mechanically ventilated patients: validity and reliability of the confusion assessment method for the intensive care unit (CAM-ICU). *JAMA.* 2001 Dec 5;286(21):2703–10.
3. Sessler CN, Gosnell MS, Grap MJ, et al. The Richmond Agitation-Sedation Scale: validity and reliability in adult intensive care unit patients. *AM J Respir Crit Care Med.* 2002;166:1338–44.
4. Randolph C, Tierney MC, Mohr E, Chase TN. The Repeatable Battery for the Assessment of Neuropsychological Status (RBANS): preliminary clinical validity. *J Clin Exp Neuropsychol.* 1998;20:310–9.

5. Reitan RM, Wolfson D. The Halstead Reitan neuropsychological test battery. Tucson AZ: Neuropsychology Press, 1985.

6. Haenggi M, Blum S, Brechbuehl R, Brunello A, Jakob SM, Takala J. Effect of sedation level on the prevalence of delirium when assessed with CAM-ICU and ICDSC. *Intensive Care Med.* 2013 Dec;39(12):2171–79.

7. Iwashyna TJ, Ely EW, Smith DM, Langa KM. Long-term cognitive impairment and functional disability among survivors of severe sepsis. *JAMA.* 2010 Oct 27;304(16):1787–94.

8. Kamdar BB, King LM, Collop NA, et al. The effect of a quality improvement intervention on perceived sleep quality and cognition in a medical ICU. *Crit Care Med.* 2013 Mar;41(3):800–9.

18

Cerebral Perfusion Pressure

Cerebral perfusion pressure management can serve as the primary goal in the treatment of traumatic intracranial hypertension with substantially improved mortality and morbidity following TBI.

—Rosner et al.[1]

Research Question: Does management of cerebral perfusion pressure (CPP) as the primary goal of therapy yield lower mortality and higher Glasgow Outcome Scale (GOS) scores than that achieved with traditional, intracranial pressure (ICP)-based techniques?

Funding: US Department of Health and Human Services, Centers for Disease Control and Prevention, National Center for Injury Prevention and Control.

Year Study Published: 1995.

Study Location: University of Alabama at Birmingham, Birmingham, Alabama.

Who Was Studied: Traumatic brain injury (TBI) patients older than 14 years admitted to the hospital with postresuscitation Glasgow Coma Scale (GCS) scores of 7 or below who did not follow commands within 24 hours. Clinical cases with hypoxemia, traumatic asphyxia, hypotension, and multiple systemic injuries were specifically included.

How Many Patients: 158.

Study Overview: See Figure 18.1 for an overview of the study's design.

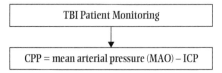

Figure 18.1 Summary of the study design.

Study Intervention: Study patients were closely monitored and managed to maintain a minimum CPP of at least 70 mm Hg, achieved using vascular volume expansion, cerebrospinal fluid drainage, systemic vasopressors (phenylephrine or norepinephrine), and mannitol. The CPP threshold value of 70 mm Hg was increased to 80 or 90+ mm Hg in certain patients if parameters indicated that the patient would benefit from a higher CPP.

All patients underwent monitoring for central venous pressure (CVP) and intra-arterial blood pressure as well as ICP through frontal ventriculostomy catheters. All patients were intubated and minute ventilation adjusted to maintain a targeted $Paco_2$ of 35 mm Hg. The goal of fluid management was to establish and maintain euvolemia to moderate hypervolemia (pulmonary capillary wedge pressures of 12 to 15 mm Hg or CVP of 8 to 10 mm Hg). CPP was calculated as the arithmetic difference of the mean arterial pressure (MAP) and the mean ICP. CSF drainage was used whenever CPP dropped below the 70 mm Hg set point; if CSF drainage was insufficient to maintain CPP at target levels, vasopressors were added. Barbiturates, hyperventilation, and hypothermia were not used.

Follow-Up: 10.5 months.

Endpoints: Mortality and outcome quality of the survivors, as measured by the GOS.

RESULTS

- The patient outcomes observed in this analysis using this CPP-based management protocol are significantly better than the outcomes observed in other reported series (Traumatic Coma Data Bank [TCDB]) using traditional ICP-based management techniques with respect to death rates, survival vs. dead or vegetative, or favorable verses nonfavorable outcome classifications.
- The average postresuscitation GCS score was 5, with the majority of patients being injured in automobile collisions, assaults, and falls.

- The overall mortality was 29%, and mortality ranged from 52% of patients with a GCS of 3 on admission to 12% of those with a GCS score of 7 on admission.
- For patients who survived, the likelihood of their having a favorable recovery was approximately 80%.
- Favorable outcomes (GOS of 4 or 5, denoting mild or moderate disability) ranged from 35% of patients with a GCS score of 3 on admission to 75% of those with a GCS score of 7 on admission.
- Only 2% of the patients in the series remained vegetative.

Criticisms and Limitations: This series of patients had an overall lower incidence of pupillary abnormalities and lower rates of surgical mass lesions. Direct comparisons between the TCDB and this series by GCS scores was not possible because the TCDB series included patients with GCS scores of 8, 9, and above.

Other Relevant Studies and Information:

- Mannitol and hypertonic saline are agents used to lower ICP. A systematic review published in 2016 reported that clinically important differences in mortality, neurologic outcomes, and ICP reduction were not observed between mannitol and hypertonic saline in the management of severe TBI. Hypertonic saline did appear to lead to fewer ICP treatment failures.[2]
- The 2017 Guidelines for the Management of Severe Traumatic Brain Injury state that "treating ICP > 22 mm Hg is recommended because values above this level are associated with increased mortality" and "the recommended target CPP value for survival and favorable outcomes is between 60 and 70 mm Hg." (Level IIb recommendations.)[3]

Summary and Implications: This study analyzing patients with TBI who underwent monitoring using CPP, rather than the standard ICP-based monitoring, demonstrated lower rates of mortality and improved outcomes compared with other analyses of patients receiving standard ICP-based monitoring. However, because this was not a controlled study, it is not possible to draw firm conclusions. Current guidelines do not recommend one type of monitoring over another but do provide thresholds for blood pressure, ICP, CPP, and advanced cerebral monitoring.

CLINICAL CASE: TBI AND MONITORING

Case History

A 47-year-old man with TBI presents for repair of a lower extremity fracture. The patient was admitted to the hospital 1 week earlier with a GCS score of 7 following a motorcycle collision. Both ICP and CPP are monitored in this patient. During the surgical procedure, the patient's ICP remains below 22 mm Hg, but his CPP declines to 50 mm Hg. What are the recommendations for managing this patient's CPP?

Suggested Answer

Current neurosurgical guidelines recommend a target CPP value between 60 and 70 mm Hg. Raising this patient's systolic blood pressure with fluids or vasopressors to at least 60 mm Hg is recommended.

References

1. Rosner MJ, Rosner SD, Johnson AH. Cerebral perfusion pressure: management protocol and clinical results. J Neurosurg. 1995 Dec;83(6):949–62.
2. Burgess S, Abu-Laban RB, Slavik RS, Vu EN, Zed PJ. A systematic review of randomized controlled trials comparing hypertonic sodium solutions and mannitol for traumatic brain injury: implications for emergency department management. Ann Pharmacother. 2016 Apr;50(4):291–300.
3. Carney N, Totten AM, O'Reilly C, et al. Guidelines for the management of severe traumatic brain injury, fourth edition. Neurosurgery. 2017 Jan 1;80(1):6–15.

Critical Care

19

An Intervention to Decrease Catheter-Related Bloodstream Infections in the Intensive Care Unit

As part of the Michigan statewide patient-safety initiative, we implemented a simple and inexpensive intervention to reduce [catheter-related bloodstream infections] in 103 ICUs. Coincident with the intervention, the median rate of infection decreased from 2.7 per 1000 catheter-days at baseline to 0 within the first 3 months after the implementation of the intervention.

—Pronovost et al.[1]

Research Question: Can rates of catheter-related bloodstream infections be reduced by implementing a safety initiative involving five simple infection-control measures by intensive care unit (ICU) staff?[1]

Sponsor: The US Agency for Healthcare Research and Quality.

Year Study Began: 2003.

Year Study Published: 2006.

Study Location: 103 intensive care units in 67 Michigan hospitals.

Who Was Studied: Patients from 103 intensive care units in 67 Michigan hospitals, representing 85% of all ICU beds in Michigan. ICUs included medical, surgical, cardiac, neurologic, surgical trauma units, and one pediatric unit.

Who Was Excluded: Data from four ICUs were excluded because these hospitals did not track the necessary data, and data from one ICU were merged and included with data from another ICU. In addition, 34 hospitals in Michigan chose not to participate in the project.

How Many Patients: A total of 375,757 catheter days, which refers to the total number of days in which catheters were in place for all study patients. For example, a patient with a catheter in place for 7 days would represent 7 catheter days.

Study Overview: As part of the Michigan Keystone ICU project, participating ICUs implemented a series of patient-safety interventions including the use of a daily goals sheet to improve staff communication, a program to improve the culture of safety among staff, and an intervention to reduce the rate of catheter-related bloodstream infections. This analysis focuses on the intervention aimed at preventing catheter-related bloodstream infections.

Rates of bloodstream infections in participating ICUs were monitored for a 3-month period before implementation of the safety initiative and for an 18-month period afterward.

Study Intervention: In preparation for implementation of the safety initiative, each ICU designated at least one physician and one nurse as team leaders. Team leaders received training in the "science of safety" and on the components of the initiative through "conference calls every other week, coaching by research staff, and statewide meetings twice a year." The team leaders, along with each hospital's infection-control staff, led implementation of the safety initiative at their respective institutions.

The safety initiative involved the promotion of five simple measures for preventing bloodstream infections:

- Hand washing
- Using sterile drapes during the insertion of central venous catheters
- Cleaning the skin with chlorhexidine disinfectant before catheter insertion

- Avoiding the femoral site for central line insertion whenever possible
- Removing unnecessary catheters

These practices were encouraged in the following ways:

- Clinicians received education about the harms of bloodstream infections and the importance of following infection-control measures.
- A cart was created in each ICU with the necessary supplies for central line insertion.
- The central line carts included a checklist reminding staff to follow the preventive measures, and clinicians were instructed to complete the checklists whenever they placed central lines.
- During daily ICU rounds, teams discussed the removal of unnecessary catheters.
- Clinician teams received regular feedback on the rates of bloodstream infections among their patients.
- ICU staff were empowered to stop central line insertion if they observed that the preventive measures were not being followed (i.e., nurses and other staff had the authority to stop doctors who were not following the safety measures).

Follow-Up: 18 months.

Endpoints: Change in the rate of catheter-related bloodstream infections before and after the initiative began.

RESULTS

- The percentage of hospital ICUs stocking chlorhexidine in central line kits increased from 19% before the start of the initiative to 64% 6 weeks afterward.
- Mean infection rates decreased continuously throughout the study period; that is, the safety initiative became increasingly more effective throughout the study period (Table 19.1).
- The safety initiative was effective among both teaching and nonteaching hospitals, as well as among both large (≥200 beds) and small (<200 beds) hospitals, though it appeared to be slightly more effective at small hospitals.

TABLE 19.1. KEY FINDINGS FROM THE KEYSTONE ICU PROJECT

Time	Median Infections per 1,000 Catheter Days at Study Hospitals*	Range of Infection Rates per 1,000 Catheter Days at Study Hospitals[†]	P Value for Comparison with Baseline Rates
Baseline	2.7	0.6–4.8	–
During implementation	1.6	0.0–4.4	≤0.05
After implementation			
0–3 months	0	0.0–3.0	≤0.002
16–18 months	0	0.0–2.4	≤0.002

*Catheter days refer to the total number of days in which catheters were in place for all study patients. For example, a patient with a catheter in place for 7 days would represent 7 catheter days.
[†]The highest and lowest infection rates among study hospitals.

Criticisms and Limitations: Because there were no control ICUs that did not implement the safety initiative, it is not possible to prove that the initiative—rather than other factors—was responsible for the observed reduction in infections. The fact that infection rates didn't decrease substantially in other states during the same time period argues against an alternative explanation, however.

It is possible that the number of reported infections during the study period decreased simply because hospital staff changed the way that they diagnosed catheter-related bloodstream infections. For example, hospital staff may have underreported these infections during the study period simply because they knew that infection rates were being closely tracked. The authors believe this is unlikely, however, because "infection rates were collected and reported" according to prespecified criteria by "hospital infection-control practitioners who were independent of the ICU staff."

It is not known how well ICU staff followed each component of the initiative, nor is it known which component was most important for reducing infection rates. For example, it is possible that most of the observed benefit resulted from a single component of the initiative such as the use of chlorhexidine disinfectant.

Finally, it is not known how much time, effort, and cost each ICU had to invest to comply with the intervention. Resource utilization was likely modest, however, because the intervention was simple and did not require expensive equipment or supplies.

Other Relevant Studies and Information:

- A follow-up analysis showed that the reduction in catheter-related bloodstream infections in Michigan was sustained for an additional 18 months (total follow-up of 36 months).[2]
- A follow-up analysis also showed that implementation of the safety initiative was associated with a reduction in all-cause ICU mortality among Medicare patients in Michigan compared with the surrounding states.[3]
- A cost analysis examining data from six hospitals that were part of the Keystone ICU Project suggested that the intervention saved money for the health care system: the average cost of the intervention was $3,375 per infection averted; however, catheter-related bloodstream infections typically cost approximately $12,000–$54,000 to treat.[4]
- The model used in the Keystone ICU initiative has been successfully implemented in other states, including Rhode Island[5] and Hawaii.[6]
- Simple checklist protocols to reduce complication rates among surgical patients have also proved highly effective.[7,8]
- Studies have suggested that the rates of other hospital-acquired infections such ventilator-associated pneumonia can be greatly reduced with the use of simple checklist protocols.[9,10]
- Despite the successes of these safety initiatives, many hospitals in the United States and around the world do not consistently use these simple measures.

Summary and Implications: Implementation of a safety initiative involving five simple infection-control measures by ICU staff was associated with a substantial reduction in catheter-related bloodstream infections. While it is not certain that the safety initiative—rather than other factors—was responsible for the observed reduction, the study provides strong evidence that this safety initiative should be implemented widely.

CLINICAL CASE: REDUCING CATHETER-RELATED BLOODSTREAM INFECTIONS IN THE INTENSIVE CARE UNIT

Case History

You are the Chief Medical Officer at a community hospital. Your hospital has a small ICU with 10 beds. Based on the results of this study, should you implement the infection-control program used in this study?

Suggested Answer

This study suggests that implementation of a safety initiative involving five simple infection-control measures by ICU staff was associated with a substantial reduction in catheter-related bloodstream infections. However, implementation of a similar program at your hospital will require an investment of staff time and resources. In addition, the program may not work as effectively at your hospital as it did in the Michigan hospitals involved in this study.

As the Chief Medical Officer, you must decide whether the investment is worth it or whether the resources could be used in better ways (e.g., to hire more clinical staff). Many experts believe that implementation of the safety initiative used in this study would be a good investment because the program is relatively inexpensive and seems to substantially reduce infections—which are not only harmful to patients but also expensive to treat. However, as Chief Medical Officer you must ultimately make this decision based on your judgment.

References

1. Pronovost P, Needham D, Berenholtz S, et al. An intervention to decrease catheter-related bloodstream infections in the ICU. *N Engl J Med*. 2006;355(26):2725–32.
2. Pronovost PJ, Goeschel CA, Colantuoni E, et al. Sustaining reductions in catheter related bloodstream infections in Michigan intensive care units: observational study. *BMJ*. 2010;340:c309.
3. Lipitz-Snyderman A, Steinwachs D, Needham DM, et al. Impact of a statewide intensive care unit quality improvement initiative on hospital mortality and length of stay: retrospective comparative analysis. *BMJ*. 2011;342:d219.
4. Waters HR, Korn R, JR, Colantuoni E, et al. The business case for quality: economic analysis of the Michigan Keystone Patient Safety Program in ICUs. *Am J Med Qual*. 2011;26(5):333–39.
5. DePalo VA, McNicoll L, Cornell M, et al. The Rhode Island ICU collaborative: a model for reducing central line-associated bloodstream infection and ventilator-associated pneumonia statewide. *Qual Saf Health Care*. 2010;19(6):555–61.
6. Lin DM, Weeks K, Bauer L, et al. Eradicating central line-associated bloodstream infections statewide: the Hawaii experience. *Am J Med Qual*. 2012;27(2):124–29.
7. Haynes AB, Weiser TG, Berry WR, et al. A surgical safety checklist to reduce morbidity and mortality in a global population. *N Engl J Med*. 2009;360:491–99.
8. de Vries EN, Prins HA, Crolla RM, et al. Effect of a comprehensive surgical safety system on patient outcomes. *N Engl J Med*. 2010 363;20:1928–37.

9. Bouadma L, Deslandes E, Lolom I, et al. Long-term impact of a multifaceted prevention program on ventilator-associated pneumonia in a medical intensive care unit. *Clin Infect Dis.* 2010;51(10):1115.

10. Berenholtz SM, Pham JC, Thompson DA, et al. Collaborative cohort study of an intervention to reduce ventilator-associated pneumonia in the intensive care unit. *Infect Control Hosp Epidemiol.* 2011;32(4):305.

20

Early Goal-Directed Therapy in the Treatment of Severe Sepsis and Septic Shock

> [Goal-directed therapy aimed at restoring] a balance between oxygen de-livery and oxygen demand . . . [in] the earliest stages of severe sepsis and septic shock . . . has significant short-term and long-term benefits.
>
> —RIVERS ET AL.[1]

Research Question: Does aggressive correction of hemodynamic disturbances in the early stages of sepsis improve outcomes?[1]

Funding: Henry Ford Health Systems Fund for Research and a Weatherby Healthcare Resuscitation Fellowship.

Year Study Began: 1997.

Year Study Published: 2001.

Study Location: The Henry Ford Hospital in Detroit, Michigan.

Who Was Studied: Adults presenting to the emergency department with se-vere sepsis or septic shock. To qualify, patients needed to have a suspected in-fection and at least two of four criteria for a systemic inflammatory response syndrome (SIRS) as well as a systolic blood pressure ≤90 mm Hg. Alternatively, they could have a suspected infection, at least two SIRS criteria, and a lactate level ≥4 mm/L (Table 20.1).

Table 20.1. SIRS CRITERIA

Temperature	$\leq 36°$ C or $\geq 38°$ C
Heart rate	≥ 90 beats/min
Respiratory rate	≥ 20 or $Paco_2$ <32 mm Hg
White cell count	$\geq 12,000$ or $\leq 4,000$ or $\geq 10\%$ bands

Who Was Excluded: Patients who were pregnant and those with any of several acute conditions, including stroke, acute coronary syndrome, acute pulmonary edema, status asthmaticus, or gastrointestinal bleeding. Patients with a contraindication to central venous catheterization were also excluded.

How Many Patients: 263.

Study Overview: See Figure 20.1 for an overview of the study's design.

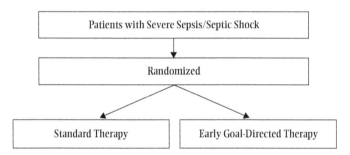

Figure 20.1 Summary of the trial design.

Study Intervention: Patients in the standard therapy group received immediate critical care consultation and were admitted to the intensive care unit as quickly as possible. Subsequent management was at the discretion of the critical care team, which was given a protocol advocating the following hemodynamic goals:

- Crystalloid in 500-mL boluses should be given every 30 minutes as needed to achieve a central venous pressure (CVP) of 8–12 mm Hg.
- Vasopressors should be used as needed to maintain a mean arterial pressure (MAP) ≥ 65 mm Hg.
- Urine output goal ≥ 0.5 mL/kg/h.

Patients in the early goal-directed therapy group were managed according to a similar protocol, but they also received central venous oxygen saturation ($Scvo_2$) monitoring from a specialized central line catheter:

- If the Scvo$_2$ was <70%, red cells were transfused to achieve a hematocrit ≥30%.
- If the transfusion was ineffective, dobutamine was given as tolerated.

In addition, and perhaps most important, patients in the early goal-directed therapy group received 6 hours of aggressive treatment *immediately* on presentation to the emergency department.

Follow-Up: 60 days.

Endpoints: Primary outcome: in-hospital mortality.

RESULTS

- During the first 6 hours, patients in the early goal-directed therapy group received more fluid, more blood transfusions, and more inotropic support than did patients in the standard therapy group.
- During the first 6 hours, patients in the early goal-directed group had higher average MAPs and a higher average Scvo$_2$; in addition, a higher proportion achieved the combined goals for CVP, MAP, and urine output.
- During the period from 7 to 72 hours, patients in the early goal-directed therapy group had better hemodynamic parameters and required less fluid, red cell transfusions, vasopressors, and mechanical ventilation.
- Mortality was lower in the early goal-directed therapy group (Table 20.2)

Table 20.2. SUMMARY OF THE TRIAL'S KEY FINDINGS

Outcome	Standard Therapy Group	Early Goal-Directed Therapy Group	P Value
Hospital length of stay*	18.4 days	14.6 days	0.04
60-day mortality	56.9%	44.3%	0.03
In-hospital mortality	46.5%	30.5%	0.009

*Among patients who survived to hospital discharge.

Criticisms and Limitations: The early goal-directed protocol involved several interventions, and therefore it is not possible to know which of these measures were most important for improving outcomes. In particular, some experts have questioned the importance of aggressive red cell transfusions and dobutamine administration based on $Scvo_2$ measurements.

Other Relevant Studies and Information:

- A trial comparing hemodynamic monitoring with $Scvo_2$ measurements vs. lactate clearance in patients with sepsis suggested that the two forms of monitoring are equivalent.[2]

Summary and Implications: Most patients with severe sepsis or septic shock should be managed with aggressive hemodynamic monitoring and support immediately on presentation in the emergency department (or, if this is not possible, in the intensive care unit) for 6 hours or until there is resolution of hemodynamic disturbances.

CLINICAL CASE: EARLY GOAL-DIRECTED THERAPY

Case History

A 48-year-old previously healthy man presents reporting that he "feels miserable." Over the past day, he has had a cough with thick green sputum as well as subjective fevers and fatigue. The symptoms worsened 2 hours before presentation, and he now has rigors, increasing fatigue, and mild to moderate dyspnea. On exam, his temperature is 39° C, his heart rate is 126 beats per minute, his respiratory rate is 24 breaths per minute, and his blood pressure is 96/64 mm Hg. His laboratory results are notable for a white blood cell count of 18,000 with 40% bands and a lactate of 3 mm/L. His chest radiograph shows a right middle lobe consolidation.

After reading this trial about early goal-directed therapy, how would you treat this patient on presentation to the emergency department?

Suggested Answer

This patient fulfills more than two SIRS criteria and has a suspected infection (pneumonia). However, he doesn't quite fulfill the criteria for severe sepsis specified in the trial because his systolic blood pressure is >90 mm Hg and his lactate level is <4 mm/L. If he did meet the criteria for severe sepsis, he should be treated immediately (in the emergency department if possible) with early goal-directed therapy:

- Crystalloid in 500-mL boluses every 30 minutes for a target CVP of 8–12 mm Hg
- Vasopressors to maintain an MAP ≥65 mm Hg
- Urine output goal ≥0.5 mL/kg/h
- Hemodynamic monitoring with $Scvo_2$ measurements (or lactate clearance measurements) and red cell transfusions followed by cautious dobutamine administration to achieve the hemodynamic goals

Even though this patient does not quite fulfill the criteria for severe sepsis, it might still be reasonable to implement early goal-directed therapy because he is so close to meeting the criteria. At the very least, he should be closely monitored and early goal-directed therapy instituted immediately if his systolic blood pressure drops below 90 mm Hg or his lactate level rises above 4 mm/L.

References

1. Rivers E, Nguyen B, Havistad S, et al. Early goal-directed therapy in the treatment of severe sepsis and septic shock. *N Engl J Med.* 2001;345(19):1368–77.
2. Jones AE, Shapiro NI, Trzeciak S, et al. Lactate clearance vs central venous oxygen saturation as goals of early sepsis therapy: a randomized clinical trial. *JAMA.* 2010;303(8):739–46.

Intensive Insulin Therapy and Pentastarch Resuscitation in Sepsis

> The use of intensive insulin therapy placed critically ill patients with sepsis at an increased risk for serious adverse events related to hypoglycemia. As used in this study, [pentastarch] was harmful, and its toxicity increased with accumulating doses.
>
> —BRUNKHORST ET AL.[1]

Research Question: What are the safety and efficacy of intensive insulin therapy compared with conventional therapy and hydroxyethyl starch (HES) compared with Ringer's lactate in patients with severe sepsis or septic shock?

Funding: German Federal Ministry of Education and Research, B. Braun, HemoCue, and Novo Nordisk.

Year Study Began: 2003.

Year Study Published: 2008.

Study Location: 18 academic tertiary hospitals in Germany.

Who Was Studied: Adult patients in multidisciplinary intensive care units (ICUs) with severe sepsis or septic shock (time of onset less than 24 hours before

admission to the ICU or less than 12 hours after admission if the condition developed in the ICU).

Who Was Excluded: Patients younger than 18 years and those who had received
more than 1,000 mL of HES in the 24 hours before randomization.

How Many Patients: 537.

Study Overview: See Figure 21.1 for an overview of the study's design.

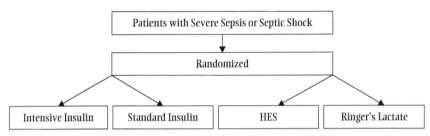

Figure 21.1 Summary of the study design.

Study Intervention: This multicenter, two-by-two factorial trial randomly
assigned patients to receive either intensive insulin therapy or conventional insulin therapy and either 10% pentastarch (a low-molecular-weight HES (200/
0.5) or Ringer's lactate. In the conventional insulin therapy group, a continuous insulin infusion was started when blood glucose level exceeded 200 mg/
dL and adjusted to maintain blood glucose levels between 180 and 200 mg/
dL; in the intensive-therapy group, insulin infusions were started when blood
glucose levels exceeded 110 mg/dL and adjusted to maintain blood glucose
levels between 80 and 110 mg/dL. Blood glucose levels were measured at
intervals of 1 to 4 hours. For fluid resuscitation, management in the Ringer's
lactate and HES groups was guided by hemodynamic target values (e.g., central venous pressure ≥8 mm Hg). Morbidity was measured by the mean score
on the Sequential Organ Failure Assessment (SOFA), a scale ranging from 0
to 4 for each of six organ systems with higher scores indicative of more severe
organ dysfunction.

Follow-Up: 90 days.

Endpoints: Primary outcomes: mortality at 28 days and morbidity (measured by SOFA). Secondary outcomes: mortality at 90 days, rate of acute renal
failure (defined as doubling of baseline serum creatinine level or the need for
renal-replacement therapy), time to hemodynamic stabilization, frequency of

vasopressor therapy, mean SOFA subscores, need for red cell transfusion, duration of mechanical ventilation, and length of ICU stay. The occurrence of severe hypoglycemia (defined as blood glucose level ≤40 mg/dL) was a safety endpoint.

RESULTS

- The trial was stopped early for safety reasons because of a significantly increased incidence of hypoglycemic events in the intensive insulin therapy group and renal failure in the HES group.
- For insulin therapy, 98.7% of patients in the intensive-therapy group received insulin on at least one study day compared with 74.1% in the conventional-therapy group, with lower mean morning blood glucose levels and higher median insulin doses per patient per day in the intensive-therapy group ($P < 0.001$ for all).
- The rate of severe hypoglycemia was higher in the intensive insulin therapy group than in the conventional-therapy group (17% vs. 4.1%, $P < 0.001$), as was the rate of serious adverse events[2] (10.9% vs. 5.2%, $P = 0.01$). Hypoglycemic episodes were more often classified as life-threatening and required prolonged hospitalization in the intensive-therapy group compared with the conventional-therapy group ($P = 0.05$).
- For insulin therapy, mortality, SOFA scores (mean or subscores), and secondary endpoints did not significantly differ between study groups. A Cox regression analysis identified the patient's APACHE II score, an age ≥60 years, and hypoglycemia as risk factors for mortality, but intensive insulin therapy was not an independent risk factor.
- For fluid resuscitation, median central venous pressure and median central venous oxygen saturation were higher in the HES group compared with the Ringer's lactate group. Hemodynamic target values were achieved faster in patients receiving HES.
- The HES group had a higher rate of acute renal failure (34.9% vs. 22.8%, $P = 0.002$), more days on which renal replacement therapy was required (18.3% vs. 9.2%), and lower median platelet counts ($P < 0.001$) and received more units of packed red blood cells than the Ringer's lactate group.
- Post hoc univariate analysis showed a direct correlation between the cumulative dose of HES received and both the need for renal replacement therapy and mortality at 90 days.

Criticisms and Limitations: This study was stopped early for safety reasons. The dose limit for HES (20 mL/kg/day) was exceeded by more than 10% on at least 1 day in 38% of patients in the HES group.

Other Relevant Studies and Information:

- The Surviving Sepsis Campaign: International Guidelines for Management of Sepsis and Septic Shock: 2016 recommend commencing insulin dosing when two consecutive blood glucose levels are >180 mg/dL. This approach should target an upper blood glucose level ≤180 mg/dL rather than an upper target blood glucose level ≤110 mg/dL (strong recommendation, high quality of evidence). The guidelines recommend against using HES for intravascular volume replacement in patients with sepsis or septic shock (strong recommendation, high quality of evidence).[3]
- A randomized, open-label, controlled trial with blinded endpoint assessment of 400 adults (with and without diabetes) undergoing on-pump cardiac surgery demonstrated that intensive intraoperative insulin therapy did not reduce perioperative death or morbidity. More deaths (four vs. zero; $P = 0.061$) and strokes (eight vs. one; $P = 0.020$) occurred in the intensive insulin treatment group.[4]

Summary and Implications: This study demonstrated that critically ill patients did not benefit from intensive insulin therapy targeting blood glucose levels of 80–110 mg/dL vs. conventional insulin therapy, nor from fluid resuscitation with HES vs. Ringer's lactate. Neither intensive insulin therapy nor fluid resuscitation with HES is currently recommended in major sepsis guidelines.

CLINICAL CASE: PERIOPERATIVE GLUCOSE AND FLUID MANAGEMENT IN SEPSIS

Case History

A 62-year-old man with sepsis comes to the operating room emergently for abdominal surgery for bowel perforation. The patient is hypotensive, and an intraoperative arterial blood gas analysis shows a blood glucose level of 149 mg/dL. Should insulin be administered to treat the patient's hyperglycemia intraoperatively? Should HES be used for fluid resuscitation?

Suggested Answer

Insulin for the treatment of hyperglycemia is not indicated at this time. The patient's blood glucose level should be monitored closely. HES should be avoided in the setting of sepsis.

References

1. Brunkhorst FM, Engel C, Bloos F, et al. Intensive insulin therapy and pentastarch resuscitation in severe sepsis. *N Engl J Med.* 2008 Jan 10;358(2):125–39.
2. What is a serious adverse event? Rockville, MD: MedWatch, FDA Safety Information and Adverse Event Reporting Program, 2004. (Accessed December 14, 2007, at http://www.fda.gov/medwatch/report/DESK/advevnt.htm.)
3. Rhodes A, Evans LE, Alhazzani W, et al. Surviving sepsis campaign: international guidelines for management of sepsis and septic shock: 2016. *Crit Care Med.* 2017 Mar;45(3):486–552.
4. Gandhi GY, Nuttall GA, Abel MD, et al. Intensive intraoperative insulin therapy versus conventional glucose management during cardiac surgery: a randomized trial. *Ann Intern Med.* 2007 Feb 20;146(4):233–43.

22

Transfusion Requirements in Critical Care (TRICC)

Our findings indicate that the use of a threshold for red-cell transfusion as low as 7.0 [grams] of hemoglobin per deciliter . . . was at least as effective as and possibly superior to a liberal transfusion [threshold of 10.0 g/dL] in critically ill patients.

—HÉBERT ET AL.[1]

Research Question: When should patients in the intensive care unit (ICU) with anemia receive red cell transfusions?[1]

Funding: The Medical Research Council of Canada and an unrestricted grant from the Bayer Company (the Bayer grant was given after funding had been secured from the Medical Research Council of Canada).

Year Study Began: 1994.

Year Study Published: 1999.

Study Location: 25 intensive care units in Canada.

Who Was Studied: Adults in medical and surgical intensive care units with a hemoglobin (Hgb) <9 g/dL who were clinically euvolemic.

Who Was Excluded: Patients with considerable active blood loss (e.g., gastrointestinal bleeding leading to a drop in hgb of at least 3 points in the preceding

12 hours), chronic anemia (documented Hgb <9 g/dL at least 1 month before admission), and those who were pregnant.

How Many Patients: 838.

Study Overview: See Figure 22.1 for an overview of the study's design.

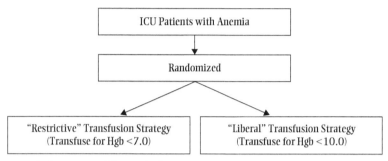

Figure 22.1 Summary of the study design.

Study Intervention: Non–leukocyte-reduced red cells were transfused according to the previous thresholds and were given 1 unit at a time. After each transfusion, the patient's hemoglobin was measured and additional transfusions were given as needed.

Follow-Up: 30 days.

Endpoints: Primary outcome: 30-day mortality. Secondary outcomes: 60-day mortality, multiorgan failure.

RESULTS

- Approximately 30% of patients had a primary respiratory diagnosis; 20% had a primary cardiac diagnosis; 15% had a primary gastrointestinal illness; and 20% had a primary diagnosis of trauma.
- Patients in the "restrictive" group received an average of 2.6 units of blood during the trial compared with an average of 5.6 units in the liberal group.
- The average daily Hgb in the "restrictive" group was 8.5 g/dL vs. 10.7 g/dL in the "liberal" group.
- As indicated in Table 22.1, there was no significant difference in 30-day mortality between patients in the "restrictive" vs. "liberal" groups; however, in a subgroup analysis involving younger and

healthier patients, 30-day mortality rates were significantly lower in the "restrictive" group.

- In another subgroup analysis involving patients with cardiac disease, there was no significant difference in 30-day mortality between patients in the "restrictive" vs. "liberal" groups; however, patients with acute coronary syndromes had nonsignificantly improved outcomes with the "liberal" transfusion strategy.[2]
- Cardiac events (pulmonary edema and myocardial infarction) were significantly more common in the "liberal" group.

Table 22.1. Summary of TRICC's Key Findings

Outcome	"Restrictive" Group	"Liberal" Group	P Value
30-day mortality	18.7%	23.3%	0.11
60-day mortality	22.7%	26.5%	0.23
Multiorgan failure*	5.3%	4.3%	0.36

*More than three failing organs.

Criticisms and Limitations: A disproportionate number of patients with severe cardiac disease did not participate in the trial because their physicians chose not to enroll them. In addition, the red cells used in this trial were not leukocyte-reduced. Some centers now routinely use leukocyte-reduced blood, which may be associated with few transfusion-related complications.

Other Relevant Studies and Information:

- A review of trials comparing restrictive vs. liberal transfusion strategies concluded that "existing evidence supports the use of restrictive transfusion [strategies] in patients who are free of serious cardiac disease"; however, "the effects of conservative transfusion [strategies] on functional status, morbidity and mortality, particularly in patients with cardiac disease, need to be tested in further large clinical trials."[3]
- Trials have supported the use of a restrictive transfusion strategy in patients undergoing elective coronary artery bypass surgery,[4] patients who have undergone surgery for a hip fracture,[5] and children in the intensive care unit.[6]
- A restrictive transfusion strategy (Hgb threshold ≤ 7 g/dL) proved superior to a liberal strategy (Hgb threshold ≤ 10 g/dL) among patients with acute upper gastrointestinal bleeding.[7]
- A small trial involving older adult patients admitted to the hospital with a hip fracture compared a liberal transfusion strategy (Hgb threshold

≤10 g/dL) with a restrictive strategy (Hgb threshold ≤8 g/dL). The trial showed lower mortality with the liberal strategy, but these findings require replication in a larger study.[8]

Summary and Implications: For most critically ill patients, waiting to transfuse red cells until the Hgb drops below 7 g/dL is at least as effective as, and likely preferable to, transfusing at an Hgb less than 10 g/dL. These findings may not apply to patients with chronic anemia, who were excluded from the trial. The results also may not apply to patients with active cardiac ischemia, who were poorly represented in the trial and had nonsignificantly worse outcomes with a transfusion threshold of 7 g/dL.

CLINICAL CASE: RED CELL TRANSFUSION IN CRITICALLY ILL PATIENTS

Case History

A 74-year-old woman with myelodysplastic syndrome is admitted to the general medicine service at your hospital with pneumonia. On review of systems, you note that she has suffered from increasing fatigue for the past 3 months. Her Hgb on admission is 8 g/dL—which has decreased from 10.5 g/dL when it was last measured 4 months ago.

Based on the results of the TRICC trial, should you give this patient a red cell transfusion?

Suggested Answer

The TRICC trial showed that, for most critically ill patients, waiting to transfuse red cells until the Hgb drops below 7 g/dL is at least as effective as, and likely preferable to, transfusing at an Hgb <10 g/dL. However, the patient in this vignette is not critically ill, and thus the results of TRICC should not be applied to her. This patient's fatigue likely results from anemia due to her myelodysplastic syndrome. Red cell transfusion would likely be appropriate for her.

References

1. Hébert PC, Wells G, Blajchman MA, et al. A multicenter, randomized, controlled clinical trial of transfusion requirements in critical care. *N Engl J Med.* 1999;340(6):409–17.

2. Hébert PC, Yetisir E, Martin C, et al. Is a low transfusion threshold safe in critically ill patients with cardiovascular diseases? *Crit Care Med.* 2001;29(2):227.

3. Carless PA, Henry DA, Carson JL, et al. Transfusion thresholds and other strategies for guiding allogeneic red blood cell transfusion. *Cochrane Database Syst Rev.* 2010;(10):CD002042.

4. Bracey AW, Radovancevic R, Riggs SA, et al. Lowering the hemoglobin threshold for transfusion in coronary artery bypass procedures: effect on patient outcome. *Transfusion.* 1999;39(10):1070.

5. Carson JL, Terrin ML, Noveck H, et al. Liberal or restrictive transfusion in high-risk patients after hip surgery. *N Engl J Med.* 2011;365(26):2453.

6. Lacroix J, Hébert PC, Hutchison JS, et al. Transfusion strategies for patients in pediatric intensive care units. *N Engl J Med.* 2007;356(16):1609–19.

7. Villanueva C, Colomo A, Bosch A, et al. Transfusion strategies for acute upper gastrointestinal bleeding. *N Engl J Med.* 2013;368(1):11–21.

8. Foss NB, Kristensen MT, Jensen PS, et al. The effects of liberal vs. restrictive transfusion thresholds on ambulation after hip fracture surgery. *Transfusion.* 2009;49(2):227.

23

Effects of Intravenous Fluid Restriction on Postoperative Complications

> The restricted perioperative intravenous fluid regimen aiming at unchanged body weight reduces complications after elective colorectal resection.
>
> —Brandstrup et al.[1]

Research Question: What are the effects of a restricted intravenous (IV) fluid regimen targeting an unchanged body weight vs. a standard regimen on complications after elective colorectal surgery?

Funding: Eastern Danish Health Science Research Forum, University of Copenhagen; Clinical Unit of Preventive Medicine and Health Promotion, H:S Bispebjerg University Hospital; The Copenhagen Hospital Corporation, Council of Research; The Danish Hospital Foundation for Medical Research, Region of Copenhagen, The Faeroe Islands and Greenland; The Danish Medical Association Research Found; The Northern Jutland Council of Research; The Research and Development Council, Vejle County; Olga Bryde Nielsens Fund; Hans and Nora Buchards Fund; Inge and Jørgen Larsen's Mindelegat; Grosserer Valdemar Foersom and wife Thyra Foersoms Fund. Nutricia A/S and N.C.

Year Study Began: 1999.

Year Study Published: 2003.

Study Location: Eight hospitals in Denmark.

Who Was Studied: ASA physical status I to III adult patients admitted for elective colorectal resection.

Who Was Excluded: Patients who were pregnant or lactating, had a history of mental disorders, language problems, excessive alcohol consumptions (greater than 35 drinks per week), diabetes mellitus, renal insufficiency, disseminated cancer, secondary cancers, inflammatory bowel disease, or diseases hindering epidural analgesia.

How Many Patients: 172.

Study Overview: See Figure 23.1 for an overview of the study's design.

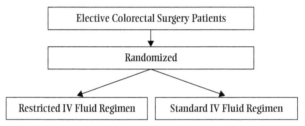

Figure 23.1 Summary of the study design.

Study Intervention: Patients receiving combined thoracic epidural and general anesthesia were randomized to two groups: the restricted fluid regimen and the standard fluid regimen. All patients were allowed clear liquids until 2 hours before surgery.

The standard group received 500 mL of normal saline to replace losses during preoperative fasting, 500 mL of hydroxyethyl starch 6% in normal saline (HAES) for volume preloading before epidural analgesia, and normal saline at a defined rate intraoperatively for replacement of insensible losses. In the restricted group, these replacements were omitted except for 500 mL of glucose 5% in water less oral fluid intake during the preoperative fast.

In the restricted group, operative blood loss was replaced on a volume-to-volume basis with HAES up to 500 mL. In contrast, in the standard group, the first 500 mL of blood loss was replaced with 1,000–1,500 mL of normal saline, and additional blood loss was replaced by HAES. Blood transfusions were initiated if blood loss approximated 1,500 mL (goal hematocrit 25%–35%). If colloid was needed after the maximum recommended dose of HAES had been reached (33 mL/kg/day), albumin 5% was administered. Urine output was not replaced.

Postoperatively, the restricted group received 1,000 mL of glucose 5% over the rest of the operative day as well as volume-to-volume replacement of drain output with HAES. In contrast, the standard group received 1,000–2,000 mL of crystalloid. Both groups were allowed to drink freely, and the restricted group received IV fluids if oral intake was inadequate, whereas the standard group received routine IV fluid therapy guided by the surgical department.

Patients in both groups were weighed preoperatively and daily for 6 days postoperatively. The restricted group received furosemide if daily weights exceeded baseline measurements by 1 kg.

All patients received nutrition through a nasoduodenal or nasojejunal feeding tube postoperatively on the day of the operation and for 3 days following.

Follow-Up: Median follow-up was 34 days postoperatively.

Endpoints: Primary outcome: complications documented within 30 days postoperatively. Secondary outcomes: death and adverse effects (including renal function impairment and postoperative hypotensive episodes).

RESULTS

- A total of 141 patients completed the trial: 69 in the restricted group and 72 in the standard group.
- Administered IV fluid volume on day of surgery was significantly less in the restricted group compared with the standard group (median 2,740 mL vs. 5,388 mL; $P < 0.0005$), but volumes of HAES administered were similar. The difference was also significant between administered IV fluid volumes on postoperative day one.
- The number of patients with postoperative complications was significantly reduced in the restricted group compared with the standard group (on intention-to-treat, per protocol, blinded and unblinded analysis). The average number of complications per patient with complications was 1.2 in the restricted group vs. 2.1 in the standard group ($P = 0.032$).
- The standard group patients had significantly higher body weights from the day of surgery to the end of measurement 6 days postoperatively.
- A dose-response relationship between complications and increasing IV fluid volumes ($P < 0.001$) as well as increasing body weight ($P < 0.001$) on the day of surgery was found to be independent of allocation group.
- Four patients died in the standard group, but no deaths occurred in the restricted group ($P = 0.12$). Causes of death: pulmonary edema,

pneumonia with septicemia, and pulmonary embolism. The deaths occurred at different institutions.

- The number of patients with a postoperative hypotensive episode was similar in the two groups, suggesting that IV fluid administration was inefficient at preventing hypotension caused by epidural analgesia.
- There was no significant difference in urinary output or serum creatinine on postoperative days 1 to 6. There was a significant difference in the number of patients with low urinary output (<0.5 mL/kg/h) on the day of surgery (3% vs. 12%; $P = 0.008$) and serum creatinine on arrival to the recovery room (mean 75.8 μmol/L vs. 86 μmol/L; $P = 0.002$) in the standard group vs. the restricted group. One case of renal failure was observed in the standard regimen group after sepsis.

Criticisms and Limitations: Deviations from the regimens were observed on the day of surgery: 15% of patients in the restricted regimen group received more IV fluid and 24% of patients in the standard group received less IV fluid than planned by protocol.

Other Relevant Studies and Information:

- At the time of this study, it was already established that perioperative fluid management in major surgery resulted in significant associated weight gain. Furthermore, such fluid overload was associated with increased hospital length of stay and complications such as increases in ventilator dependence and time to return of bowel function.[2,3]
- A randomized clinical trial published in 2012 comparing extreme fluid restriction to a standard fast-track protocol in colorectal surgery found no difference in primary hospital stay or stay including readmission days. The proportion of patients with complications was significantly lower in the restricted regimen group compared with the standard regimen group (31 of 79 vs. 47 of 82; $P = 0.027$). Vasopressors were more often required in the restricted regimen group (97% vs. 80%; $P < 0.001$).[4]
- The 2013 Enhanced Recovery After Surgery (ERAS®) Society Guidelines for Perioperative Care in Elective Colonic Surgery recommend goal-directed fluid therapy with balanced crystalloid solutions. Vasopressors should be considered for intraoperative and

postoperative management of epidural-induced hypotension provided the patient is normovolemic.[5]

Summary and Implications: This randomized, observer-blinded clinical trial demonstrated that a restricted IV fluid regimen aimed at unchanged body weight reduced complications after elective colorectal surgery.

CLINICAL CASE: PERIOPERATIVE FLUID MANAGEMENT

Case History

A 55-year-old man with colon cancer presents for laparotomy and resection under general anesthesia with a thoracic epidural for postoperative pain management. The patient has a history of hypertension and coronary artery disease. What are the perioperative fluid management goals and strategies to achieve them?

Suggested Answer

The benefits of maintaining perioperative euvolemia and avoiding excessive weight gain from IV fluid administration in colorectal surgery has been demonstrated in numerous studies. This patient should be weighed preoperatively. Careful intake and output documentation and weighing the patient daily postoperatively would help determine total fluid balance. Intraoperatively, fluid administration should be aimed at maintaining euvolemia and guided by total blood loss rather than urine output. Vasopressors rather than IV fluid boluses can be used to counteract hypotension associated with epidural analgesia.

References

1. Brandstrup B, Tønnesen H, Beier-Holgersen R, et al. Effects of intravenous fluid restriction on postoperative complications: comparison of two perioperative fluid regimens: a randomized assessor-blinded multicenter trial. *Ann Surg.* 2003 Nov;238(5):641–48.
2. Lobo DN, Bostock KA, Neal KR, Perkins AC, Rowlands BJ, Allison SP. Effect of salt and water balance on recovery of gastrointestinal function after elective colonic resection: a randomised controlled trial. *Lancet.* 2002 May 25;359(9320):1812–18.

3. Lowell JA, Schifferdecker C, Driscoll DF, Benotti PN, Bistrian BR. Postoperative fluid overload: not a benign problem. *Crit Care Med.* 1990 Jul;18(7):728–33.

4. Abraham-Nordling M, Hjern F, Pollack J, Prytz M, Borg T, Kressner U. Randomized clinical trial of fluid restriction in colorectal surgery. *Br J Surg.* 2012 Feb;99(2):186–91.

5. Gustafsson UO, Scott MJ, Schwenk W, et al. Guidelines for perioperative care in elective colonic surgery: Enhanced Recovery After Surgery (ERAS®) Society recommendations. *World J Surg.* 2013 Feb;37(2):259–84.

24

The Saline vs. Albumin Fluid Evaluation (SAFE) Study

In conclusion, our study provides evidence that albumin and saline should be considered clinically equivalent treatments for intravascular volume resuscitation in a heterogeneous population of patients in the ICU. Whether either albumin or saline confers benefit in more highly selected populations of critically ill patients requires further study.

—THE SAFE STUDY INVESTIGATORS[1]

Research Question: What is the effect of fluid resuscitation with albumin or saline on outcomes in the intensive care unit (ICU)?

Funding: Auckland District Health Board, Middlemore Hospital, Health Research Council of New Zealand, Australian Commonwealth Department of Health and Aged Care, Australian National Health and Medical Research Council, Health Department of Western Australia, New South Wales Health Department, Northern Territory Health Services, Queensland Health Services Department, Royal Hobart Hospital (Tasmania), South Australian Department of Human Services, and the Victorian Department of Human Services.

Year Study Began: 2001.

Year Study Published: 2004.

Study Location: Sixteen academic hospitals in Australia and New Zealand.

Who Was Studied: Adult patients admitted to closed, multidisciplinary ICUs who required fluid resuscitation, as judged by their treating physicians, and who had at least one of the following: heart rate >90 beats per minute; systolic blood pressure (SBP) <100 mm Hg; mean arterial pressure (MAP) <75 mm Hg or a 40 mm Hg decrease in SBP or MAP from baseline or requirement for inotropes or vasopressors to maintain blood pressure at those levels; central venous pressure (CVP) <10 mm Hg; pulmonary capillary wedge pressure <12 mm Hg; respiratory variation in SBP or MAP >5 mm Hg; capillary refill time >1 second; urine output <0.5 mL/kg for 1 hour.

How Many Patients: 6,997.

Who Was Excluded: Patients with a previous adverse reaction to human albumin, religious objection to the administration of human blood products, need for plasmapheresis, previous enrollment in the SAFE study, admission to the ICU following cardiac surgery or liver transplantation, or admission to the ICU for the treatment of burns; patients who were brain dead or judged likely to progress to brain death within 24 hours; patients unlikely to survive longer than 24 hours following eligibility assessment; patients who received previous "fluid resuscitation that was prescribed within the study ICU and during the current hospital admission"; and patients who were "transferred to the study ICU from a non-study ICU and received a fluid bolus or fluid resuscitation for the treatment of volume depletion in the non-study ICU."

Study Overview: See Figure 24.1 for an overview of the study's design.

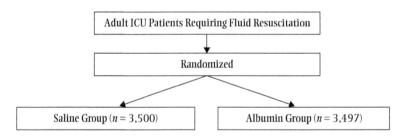

Figure 24.1 Summary of the study design.

Study Intervention: Patients were randomized to receive either 4% albumin or normal saline for intravascular fluid resuscitation for 28 days. Blinding was ensured by supplying study fluids in identical 500-mL bottles with specially designed administration sets. Monitoring (CVP, pulmonary artery catheterization) and the administration of additional fluids (maintenance, specific replacement, enteral or parenteral nutrition, and blood products) were at the discretion of the treating clinicians.

Follow-Up: Until death, ICU discharge, or a total of 28 days from enrollment.

Endpoints: Primary outcome: mortality from any cause during the 28 days following randomization. Secondary outcomes: survival time, proportion of patients who had new organ failures, duration of mechanical ventilation, duration of renal replacement therapy, and duration of ICU and hospital stay. Additionally, mortality within 28 days of randomization was examined in six predefined subgroups: the presence or absence of trauma, the presence or absence of severe sepsis, and the presence or absence of acute respiratory distress syndrome at baseline.

RESULTS

- Baseline patient characteristics were similar between the two study groups, with the only statistically significant difference being a higher mean CVP in the albumin group vs. the saline group (9.0 ± 4.7 mm Hg vs. 8.6 ± 4.6 mm Hg; $P = 0.03$).
- There was no significant difference in overall mortality, proportion of patients with new single-organ and multiple-organ failure, mean number of days spent in the ICU, days spent in the hospital, days of mechanical ventilation, or days of renal replacement therapy between the two study groups.
- Patients assigned to albumin received less fluid than patients assigned to saline during the first 4 days and a greater volume of packed red cells during the first 2 days.
- Among the six predefined subgroups, there was a trend to significance between the albumin and saline groups in death within 28 days for those patients with severe sepsis and those with trauma.
- For the trauma subgroup, the increased relative risk for death among patients with trauma compared with those without trauma resulted from an excess number of deaths among patients who had trauma with brain injury.

Criticisms and Limitations: This study was not sufficiently powered to detect small differences in mortality within the six predefined subgroups. The primary outcome of mortality within 28 days may not be the most appropriate clinical outcome for traumatic brain injury patients, who constituted only 7% of the study population; outcomes such as long-term survival and functional neurologic status may be more meaningful.

Other Relevant Studies and Information:

- In 2007, the SAFE Study Investigators published a post hoc analysis of the subgroup of patients with traumatic brain injury, further classifying patients by severity on the basis of the Glasgow Coma Scale (GCS) in which severe brain injury is defined as baseline GCS score of 3–8. Analysis of the overall brain-injured population demonstrated a significantly higher mortality and lower favorable neurologic outcomes at 24 months in the albumin group, which was attributable to differences in the severely brain-injured patients (GCS 3–8). Among patients with baseline GCS scores of 9–12, there was no significant difference between the albumin and saline groups in terms of mortality or favorable neurologic outcomes at 24 months. This analysis suggests that saline is superior to albumin for resuscitation of patients with severe traumatic brain injury.[2]
- In 2011, the SAFE Study Investigators published a post hoc analysis of the subgroup of patients with severe sepsis, with the purpose of better defining the effects of albumin or saline on specific organ function (using serial Sequential Organ Failure Assessment [SOFA] scores) in addition to mortality. Overall 28-day mortality favored albumin resuscitation with an odds ratio of 0.71 (95% confidence interval = 0.52–0.97; $P = 0.03$). There was no difference between respiratory or renal SOFA scores with the use of albumin vs. saline. There was an observed increase in hepatic SOFA scores with the use of albumin; this was felt to be secondary to the presence of bilirubin in the albumin solution rather than an indication of hepatic deterioration. Although the difference did not reach statistical significance, cardiovascular SOFA scores were lower in the albumin group, possibly attributable to higher CVP and lower heart rates in that group.[3]
- The Surviving Sepsis Campaign: International Guidelines for Management of Sepsis and Septic Shock: 2016 recommend crystalloids as the fluid of choice for initial resuscitation and subsequent intravascular volume replacement in patients with sepsis and septic shock (strong recommendation, moderate quality of evidence). Use of albumin is suggested in addition to crystalloids for initial resuscitation and subsequent intravascular volume replacement when patients

require substantial amounts of crystalloids (weak recommendation, low quality of evidence).[4]

Summary and Implications: This large, multicenter, prospective, randomized, double-blind trial failed to demonstrate a benefit of albumin vs. crystalloid solution for resuscitation in the ICU. These findings are consistent with other studies.[5,6] Post hoc analyses from the SAFE study have, however, suggested certain patient subgroups that may benefit from receiving saline over albumin (severe brain injury patients) and albumin over saline (severe sepsis patients). These findings require further validation, however.

CLINICAL CASE: FLUID RESUSCITATION IN THE ICU

Case History

A 67-year-old man is admitted to the ICU with pneumonia and sepsis. The patient is tachycardic to a heart rate of 105 beats per minute and has a SBP in the 80s. Antibiotics are promptly administered. The patient requires volume resuscitation. What is the fluid of choice for initial resuscitation? Suppose the patient receives a substantial amount of crystalloid but is requiring subsequent intravascular volume replacement; should albumin be considered?

Suggested Answer

Crystalloid is the fluid of choice for initial resuscitation and subsequent intravascular volume replacement in patients with sepsis and septic shock. The use of albumin is suggested in addition to crystalloids when patients require substantial amounts of crystalloids for initial resuscitation and subsequent intravascular volume replacement. Hydroxyethyl starch solutions should be avoided in the setting of sepsis.

References

1. The SAFE Study Investigators. A comparison of albumin and saline for fluid resuscitation in the intensive care unit. *N Engl J Med.* 2004 May 27;350(22):2247–56.
2. The SAFE Study Investigators. Saline or albumin for fluid resuscitation in patients with traumatic brain injury. *N Engl J Med.* 2007 Aug 30;357(9):874–84.
3. The SAFE Study Investigators. Impact of albumin compared to saline on organ function and mortality of patients with severe sepsis. *Intensive Care Med.* 2011 Jan;37(1):86–96.

4. Rhodes A, Evans LE, Alhazzani W, et al. Surviving sepsis campaign: international guidelines for management of sepsis and septic shock: 2016. *Crit Care Med.* 2017 Mar;45(3):486–552.

5. Cochrane Injuries Group Albumin Reviewers. Human albumin administration in critically ill patients: systematic review of randomised controlled trials. *BMJ.* 1998 Jul 25;317(7153):235–40.

6. Wilkes MM, Navickis RJ. Patient survival after human albumin administration. A meta-analysis of randomized, controlled trials. *Ann Intern Med.* 2001 Aug 7;135(3):149–64.

SECTION 5

Perioperative Medicine

25

Prevention of Intraoperative Awareness
in High-Risk Surgical Patients

The BAG-RECALL trial did not demonstrate the superiority of a [electroencephalogram-derived bispectral index] protocol over a protocol incorporating standard [end-tidal anesthetic-agent concentration] monitoring for the prevention of intraoperative awareness.

—AVIDAN ET AL.[1]

Research Question: Is the electroencephalogram-derived bispectral index (BIS) superior to standard monitoring of end-tidal anesthetic-agent concentration (ETAC) for the prevention of intraoperative awareness?

Funding: Foundation for Anesthesia Education and Research, American Society of Anesthesiologists, Winnipeg Regional Health Authority, University of Manitoba Department of Anesthesia, Department of Anesthesiology at Washington University in St. Louis, and Department of Anesthesiology at University of Chicago.

Year Study Began: 2008.

Year Study Published: 2011.

Study Location: Washington University in St. Louis, University of Chicago, and University of Manitoba.

Who Was Studied: Patients ≥18 years of age undergoing elective surgery under general anesthesia with isoflurane, sevoflurane, or desflurane who were at high risk for intraoperative awareness (requiring at least one of the following: planned open heart surgery, aortic stenosis, pulmonary hypertension, use of opiates, use of benzodiazepines, use of anticonvulsant drugs, daily alcohol consumptions, ASA physical status IV, end-stage lung disease, history of intraoperative awareness, history of or anticipated difficult intubation, cardiac ejection fraction <40%, and marginal exercise tolerance).

Who Was Excluded: Patients who had dementia, were unable to provide written informed consent, or had a history of stroke with residual neurologic deficits.

How Many Patients: 6,041.

Study Overview: See Figure 25.1 for an overview of the study's design.

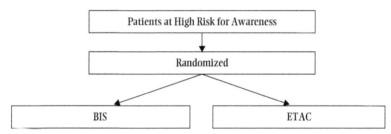

Figure 25.1 Summary of the study design.

Study Intervention: Patients at high-risk for intraoperative awareness were randomized to receive either BIS-guided or ETAC-guided general anesthesia in this prospective, multicenter, randomized, controlled trial. For each patient ETAC was monitored and a BIS Quatro (Covidien) sensor applied to the forehead. The BIS group had audible alerts if the BIS value was <40 or >60 on a scale of 0 to 100 but did not have alerts for ETAC values. Providers of patients in the ETAC group were blinded to BIS values but had audible alerts if the ETAC was <0.7 or >1.3 age-adjusted minimum alveolar concentration (MAC). BIS values and ETACs were recorded at a minimum interval of 1 minute. Both protocols included structured education and checklists. Intraoperative awareness was assessed with a modified Brice questionnaire[2] within the first 72 hours postoperatively and again at 30 days after extubation. Patients reporting intraoperative awareness were assessed by a different evaluator with additional structured questions and offered a referral to psychology. Three experts reviewed responses and classified patients into three categories: definite awareness, possible awareness, or no awareness.

Awareness was graded according to the Michigan Awareness Classification Instrument.[3]

Follow-Up: Within the first 72 hours postoperatively and at 30 days after extubation.

Endpoint: Primary outcome: incidence of definite intraoperative awareness. Secondary outcomes: incidence of definite or possible intraoperative awareness and incidence of distressing experience of awareness.

RESULTS

- A total of 5,714 patients completed at least one postoperative interview and were included in the primary analysis. There was no difference between the two study groups with respect to amount of anesthesia administered or rate of major postoperative adverse outcomes.
- A smaller percentage of patients in the ETAC group experienced intraoperative awareness compared with the BIS group, but the difference was not statistically significant.
- A total of 49 patients reported intraoperative awareness, with 9 having definite awareness (7 patients in the BIS group and 2 in the ETAC group) and 27 having definite or possible awareness. A total of 8 patients in the BIS group vs. 1 patient in the ETAC group had a distressing experience of awareness (e.g., reports of fear, anxiety, suffocation, sense of doom, or sense of impending death).
- There was a significant difference in patient characteristics between the 27 patients experiencing definite or possible intraoperative awareness compared with patients not experiencing awareness: patients with awareness met a median of one additional high-risk inclusion criteria ($P = 0.002$) and had a median of one additional preexisting medical condition ($P = 0.003$).
- A total of 5 of the 9 patients experiencing definite awareness and 6 of the 18 patients experiencing possible awareness did not have either BIS values greater than 60 or ETAC values less than 0.7 age-adjusted MAC.

Criticisms and Limitations: A number of patients were not interviewed post-operatively due to mental status or death before the initial interview; missing data could have an important effect on the results of a study examining a rare outcome. Unidentified risk factors for intraoperative awareness could have been unequally distributed between the two study groups.

Other Relevant Studies and Information:

- This study provided a counterpoint to the B-AWARE Trial (results published in 2004), which demonstrated BIS-guided anesthesia to reduce the risk for intraoperative awareness in at-risk adult surgical patients undergoing general anesthesia with the use of muscle relaxants. The B-AWARE Trial included 2,463 patients (1,225 assigned to the BIS group and 1,238 to the routine care group). There were two reports of confirmed awareness in the BIS-guided group and 11 reports in the routine care group ($P = 0.022$).[4]
- This study followed the smaller, single-center B-UNAWARE Trial (results published in 2008) of 1,941 patients (967 assigned to the BIS group and 974 to the ETAG group) and confirmed the finding that the incidence of intraoperative awareness was not reduced with BIS monitoring. In the B-UNAWARE Trial, 2 patients in each study group experienced definite intraoperative awareness, with a BIS value greater than 60 in 1 case and the ETAC less than 0.7 MAC in 3 cases.[5]

Summary and Implications: This trial failed to demonstrate the superiority of a BIS protocol over a protocol incorporating standard ETAC monitoring for the prevention of intraoperative awareness.

CLINICAL CASE: GENERAL ANESTHEISA AND AWARENESS

Case History

A 55-year-old man presents for major abdominal surgery under general anesthesia (with the use of muscle relaxants) secondary to cancer. The patient is obese (body mass index 35), has a history of hypertension and coronary artery disease, and has marginal exercise tolerance because of osteoarthritis. He reports drinking one to two beers daily. His list of medications includes a beta blocker and lorazepam, which he takes regularly for insomnia. Given this patient's past medical, social history, and planned procedure, the risk for intraoperative awareness should be addressed. How do you proceed?

Suggested Answer

Beta-blocker therapy may blunt hemodynamic changes and cause pharmacologic masking of signs of insufficient depth of anesthesia. Chronic alcohol consumption is associated with increased MAC requirements. The patient's use of benzodiazepines and marginal exercise tolerance puts him at additional risk for intraoperative awareness. Given the patient's risk factors and the need for muscle relaxants during the procedure, adequate anesthetic depth should be monitored and maintained. Intraoperative hypotension should be first treated with volume replacement or vasopressors; caution should be exercised if decreasing depth of anesthesia is necessary. A combination of sedatives and hypnotic, analgesic, and anesthetic agents could be used.

References

1. Avidan MS, Jacobsohn E, Glick D, et al. Prevention of intraoperative awareness in a high-risk surgical population. N Engl J Med. 2011 Aug 18;365(7):591–600.
2. Brice DD, Hetherington RR, Utting JE. A simple study of awareness and dreaming during anaesthesia. *Br J Anaesth*. 1970 Jun;42(6):535–42.
3. Mashour GA, Tremper KK, Avidan MS. Protocol for the "Michigan Awareness Control Study": a prospective, randomized, controlled trial comparing electronic alerts based on bispectral index monitoring or minimum alveolar concentration for the prevention of intraoperative awareness. *BMC Anesthesiol.* 2009 Nov 5;9:7.
4. Myles PS, Leslie K, McNeil J, Forbes A, Chan MT. Bispectral index monitoring to prevent awareness during anaesthesia: the B-Aware randomised controlled trial. *Lancet.* 2004 May 29;363(9423):1757–63.
5. Avidan MS, Zhang L, Burnside BA, et al. Anesthesia awareness and the bispectral index. *N Engl J Med.* 2008 Mar 13;358(11):1097–108.

26

Perioperative Medication Errors and Adverse Drug Events

Approximately one in twenty perioperative medication administrations, and every second operation, resulted in a medication error and/or adverse drug event. More than one third of these errors led to observed patient harm, and the remaining two thirds had the potential for patient harm. These rates are markedly higher than those reported by existing retrospective surveys.

—NANJI ET AL.[1]

Research Question: What are the rates, types, severity, and preventability of medication errors (MEs) and adverse drug events (ADEs) in the perioperative setting during anesthesia care?

Funding: Doctors Company Foundation and the National Institute of General Medical Sciences of the National Institutes of Health.

Year Study Began: 2013.

Year Study Published: 2016.

Study Location: Massachusetts General Hospital, Boston, Massachusetts.

Who Was Studied: Randomly selected operations.

Who Was Excluded: Anesthesia providers who were members of the study team, those performing certain types of procedures (pediatric and cardiac), and those with off-site procedural locations.

How Many Patients: 277 operations on 275 patients, with a total of 3,671 medication administrations.

Study Overview: See Figure 26.1 for an overview of the study's design.

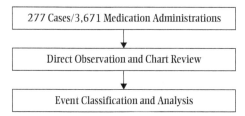

Figure 26.1 Summary of the study design.

Study Intervention: All anesthesia care providers were eligible to participate and received information about the study (with the option to opt out). Study observers underwent observer training with an emphasis on techniques used to minimize the effect of the observer on the observed (Hawthorne effect). The medication administration process was defined to involve the stages of requesting, dispensing, preparing, administering, and documenting a medication, as well as relevant monitoring. An ME was defined as "failure to complete a required action in the medication administration process, or the use of an incorrect plan or action to achieve a patient care aim." An ADE was defined as "patient harm or injury due to a medical intervention related to a drug, regardless of whether an error in the medication process occurs." Standardized data collection forms were used to document in real time all medications administered as well as any MEs and/or ADEs observed. Study cases also underwent chart review of drug dosages and vital signs. All identified events were reviewed, and events not deemed to be MEs and/or ADEs were excluded. ADE and potential for ADE severity were judged on a four-point Likert scale (significant, serious, life-threatening, and fatal), and preventability was grouped into two categories (probably preventable or probably not preventable). Each ME type was assigned to a prevention strategy believed to have the potential to reduce the likelihood of the ME and/or associated ADE.

Endpoints: Primary outcomes: the incidence of MEs and ADEs. Secondary outcomes: MEs and ADEs by patient characteristics (age, sex, race, American Society of Anesthesiologists [ASA] physical status score, body mass index [BMI], procedure type, procedure duration, and number of medication administrations).

RESULTS

- A total of 277 operations were observed with 3,671 medication administrations of which 193 (5.3%, 95% confidence interval = 4.5–6) involved an ME and/or ADE (153 MEs, 91 ADEs).
- Of the 153 MEs, 51 errors (33.3%) led to an observed ADE, and an additional 70 errors (45.8%) had the potential for patient harm.
- Of the 153 MEs, 99 (64.7%) were serious, 51 (33.3%) were significant, and 3 (2%) were life-threatening.
- Of the 193 medication administrations involving an ME and/or ADE, 153 (79.3%) were preventable and 40 (20.7%) were nonpreventable.
- Procedures lasting longer than 6 hours had higher total event rates ($P < 0.0001$), ME rates ($P < 0.0001$), and ADE rates ($P = 0.004$) than shorter procedures.
- Procedures with 13 or more medication administrations had higher event rates ($P = 0.02$) and ADE rates ($P = 0.002$) than those with 12 or fewer medication administrations.
- Event rates ($P = 0.01$), ME rates ($P = 0.03$), and ADE rates ($P = 0.02$) varied by patient race.
- The most common medication error types were labeling error, wrong dose error, and omitted medication/failure to act.

Criticisms and Limitations: This study used a broad definition for medication error types, including examples such as failure to document an intubation (documentation error) or failure to check a blood pressure before induction (monitoring error). The study was conducted at a large tertiary care academic institution with an electronic anesthesia information management system and a bar code–assisted syringe-labeling system; results may not be generalizable to nonteaching hospitals without similar technologies. The sample size may not have been large enough to detect differences in event rates by patient characteristics (e.g., ASA score, BMI, procedure type).

Other Relevant Studies and Information:

- Prior studies on anesthesia ME rates contained largely self-reported data and determined ME rates to be much lower than those reported by Nanji et al: 1 in 133 anesthetics reported by Webster et al.[2] and 1 in 274 anesthetics reported by Llewellyn et al.[3]
- Studies based on self-reporting of MEs compared with chart review or direct observation may grossly underestimate the true incidence of MEs. For example, in a study of 2,557 doses of medications administered on hospital wards, Flynn et al.[4] found 456 MEs by direct observation, 34 by chart review, and only 1 by self-report.

Summary and Implications: This prospective observational study reported that approximately 1 in 20 perioperative medication administrations, and every second operation, resulted in an ME and/or an ADE. These rates are markedly higher than those reported by prior retrospective surveys. Process- and technology-based solutions may address the root causes of MEs to reduce their incidence.

CLINICAL CASE: PERIOPERATIVE MEDICATION ERROR

Case History

A 61-year-old woman undergoing a procedure with general anesthesia is to receive ondansetron for postoperative nausea and vomiting prophylaxis. The anesthesia provider selected a vial from the ondansetron bin in the medication drawer, drew up the medication into a syringe, and administered the medication to the patient. Immediately, bradycardia is noted on the monitor. The blood pressure cuff is cycled but is reading "unable to measure systolic." On examination, the patient has bounding carotid pulses, and the electrocardiogram shows new ST depressions. The vial thought to be ondansetron is examined closely and found to be vasopressin. Nitroglycerine is administered with resolution of both hypertension and ST depressions. How should this medication error be handled?

Suggested Answer

First and foremost, the patient should be monitored and stabilized appropriately. Postoperatively, the event should be disclosed to the patient and reported to departmental or perioperative quality assurance processes. If medication errors are used to facilitate process or technology-based solutions, it is important to consider that true anesthesia medication error rates are likely significantly higher than self-reported rates.

References

1. Nanji KC, Patel A, Shaikh S, Seger DL, Bates DW. Evaluation of perioperative medication errors and adverse drug events. *Anesthesiology.* 2016 Jan;124(1):25–34.
2. Webster CS, Merry AF, Larsson L, McGrath KA, Weller J. The frequency and nature of drug administration error during anaesthesia. *Anaesth Intensive Care.* 2001 Oct;29(5):494–500.
3. Llewellyn RL, Gordon PC, Wheatcroft D, et al. Drug administration errors: a prospective survey from three South African teaching hospitals. *Anaesth Intensive Care.* 2009 Jan;37(1):93–8.
4. Flynn EA, Barker KN, Pepper GA, Bates DW, Mikeal RL. Comparison of methods for detecting medication errors in 36 hospitals and skilled-nursing facilities. *Am J Health Syst Pharm.* 2002 Mar 1;59(5):436–46.

27

Surgical Safety Checklist

Implementation of the checklist was associated with concomitant reductions in the rates of death and complications among patients at least 16 years of age who were undergoing noncardiac surgery in a diverse group of hospitals.

—HAYNES ET AL.[1]

Research Question: Does the implementation of a 19-item surgical safety checklist designed to improve team communication and consistency of care reduce complications and deaths associated with surgery?

Funding: World Health Organization (WHO).

Year Study Began: 2007.

Year Study Published: 2009.

Study Location: Eight hospitals representing a diverse set of socioeconomic environments in eight countries (Canada, India, Jordan, New Zealand, Philippines, Tanzania, Great Britain, and the United States).

Who Was Studied: Patients ≥16 years of age undergoing noncardiac surgery.

How Many Patients: 7,688.

Study Overview: See Figure 27.1 for an overview of the study's design.

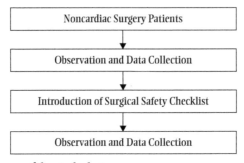

Figure 27.1 Summary of the study design.

Study Intervention: In this prospective study of preintervention and postintervention periods, baseline data on clinical processes and outcomes were collected from 3,733 consecutively enrolled patients. After the introduction of the surgical safety checklist (SSC), data on an additional 3,955 consecutively enrolled patients were collected. A local data collector represented each site after undergoing training in the identification and reporting of measures and complications. Each hospital chose between one and four operating rooms to serve as study rooms. The local study team was given information about identified deficiencies and introduced the checklist to staff with lectures, written materials, and direct guidance over a period of 1 week to 1 month; data collection resumed during the first week of checklist use. The checklist was used at three points during care: before anesthesia induction, immediately before incision, and before the patient left the operating room. Data on at least 500 consecutively enrolled patients were contributed by each study location.

Follow-Up: Until discharge or for 30 days postoperatively, whichever came first.

Endpoints: Primary outcome: occurrence of any major complication as defined by the American College of Surgeons' National Surgical Quality Improvement Program.[2] Secondary outcome: assessment of adherence to a subgroup of six safety processes included in the checklist.

RESULTS

- Analysis of patient and case characteristics between the two phases of the study did not yield any significant differences. Neither case-mix nor method of data collection (direct observation vs. unobserved clinical teams) affected the significance of the changes in rates of complications or death.

- The overall rate of complication decreased from 11% at baseline to 7% ($P < 0.001$), and in-hospital rate of death decreased from 1.5% to 0.8% ($P = 0.003$) after the introduction of the checklist. The overall rates of surgical-site infection and unplanned reoperation also declined ($P < 0.001$ and $P = 0.047$, respectively).
- All sites demonstrated a reduction in the rate of major postoperative complications, with significant reduction at three sites (one high-income location and two in lower-income locations) after checklist implementation.
- The effect of the checklist intervention remained significant on the rate of death or complications after the removal of any one site from the model.
- During the preintervention period, all six safety measures were performed for 34.2% of the patients compared with 56.7% after checklist implementation ($P < 0.001$).

Criticisms and Limitations: Data collection was restricted to inpatient complications and therefore likely underestimates total complication rates. The Hawthorne effect (an improvement in performance due to subjects' knowledge of being observed) cannot be ruled out, but data analysis demonstrated that the presence of study personnel in the operating room was not responsible for the change in complication rates after intervention. Assessment of adherence to safety measures demonstrated moderate compliance.

Other Relevant Studies and Information:

- A systematic review and meta-analysis[3] evaluated current evidence regarding the effectiveness of the SSC in reducing postoperative complications. There was heterogeneity in methodology among the seven included studies. The conclusion stated: "the evidence is highly suggestive of a reduction in postoperative complications and mortality following implementation of the WHO SSC, but cannot be regarded as definitive in the absence of higher-quality studies."
- A survey of frontline medical professionals across the globe (6,269 medical professionals from 69 countries responded) investigated attitudes and factors associated with use of the SSC. Results suggest that

the use of the SSC is variable across countries, especially in low- and middle-income countries.[4]

- In 2004, The Joint Commission enacted a Universal Protocol[5] for preventing wrong-site, wrong-procedure, and wrong-person surgery. The protocol requires performing a time out before beginning a procedure and applies to all accredited hospitals, ambulatory care, and office-based surgery facilities.

Summary and Implications: There was a reduction in the rate of major complications during hospitalization within the first 30 days postoperatively after the implementation of a 19-item SSC at eight hospitals around the world.

References

1. Haynes AB, Weiser TG, Berry WR, et al. A surgical safety checklist to re-duce morbidity and mortality in a global population. *N Engl J Med.* 2009 Jan 29;360(5):491–99.
2. Khuri SF, Daley J, Henderson W, et al. The National Veterans Administration Surgical Risk Study: risk adjustment for the comparative assessment of the quality of surgical care. *J Am Coll Surg.* 1995 May;180(5):519–31.
3. Bergs J, Hellings J, Cleemput I, et al. Systematic review and meta-analysis of the effect of the World Health Organization surgical safety checklist on postoperative complications. *Br J Surg.* 2014 Feb;101(3):150–8.
4. Vohra RS, Cowley JB, Bhasin N, Barakat HM, Gough MJ. Attitudes towards the sur-gical safety checklist and factors associated with its use: a global survey of frontline medical professionals. *Ann Med Surg* (Lond). 2015 Apr 20;4(2):119–23.
5. https://www.jointcommission.org/standards_information/up.aspx.   Accessed January 2018.

28

Prevention of Postoperative Nausea and Vomiting

Because antiemetic interventions are similarly effective and act independently, the safest or least expensive should be used first . . . and multiple interventions should be reserved for high-risk patients.

—APFEL ET AL.[1]

Research Question: What is the efficacy of six well-established prophylactic antiemetic strategies individually and in combination for the prevention of postoperative nausea and vomiting (PONV)?

Funding: Grant (1518 TG 72) from the Klinik für Anaesthesiologie, Julius-Maximilians Universität, Würzburg, Germany; a Helsinki University Central Hospital State Allocation grant (TYH 0324) from Helsinki University Central Hospital, University of Helsinki, Helsinki, Finland; AstraZeneca, Wedel, Germany; GlaxoSmithKline, Hamburg, Germany; the Gheens Foundation, Louisville, Kentucky; the Joseph Drown Foundation, Los Angeles, California; the Commonwealth of Kentucky Research Challenge Trust Fund, Louisville, Kentucky; and a Health Grant (GM 061655) from the National Institutes of Health, Bethesda, Maryland.

Year Study Began: 2000.

Year Study Published: 2004.

Study Location: 28 centers in Europe.

Who Was Studied: Adults undergoing elective surgery under general anesthesia (expected duration of at least 1 hour) who had a risk for PONV exceeding 40% based on a simplified risk score (based on the presence of at least two of the following risk factors: female sex, nonsmoker status, previous history of PONV or motion sickness, and anticipated use of postoperative opioids).

Who Was Excluded: Patients with contraindication to study medications, those who had taken emetogenic or antiemetic medication within 24 hours before surgery, those expected to require postoperative mechanical ventilation, and those pregnant or lactating.

How Many Patients: 5,199.

Study Overview: See Figure 28.1 for an overview of the study's design.

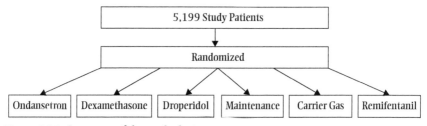

Figure 28.1 Summary of the study design.

Study Intervention: The antiemetic efficacy of six individual treatments and the combination of two or three interventions were simultaneously evaluated according to a 2^6 factorial design, yielding 64 different treatment combinations. Three of the prophylactic interventions involved an antiemetic drug (ondansetron, dexamethasone, or droperidol), and the other three consisted of using propofol instead of a volatile anesthetic, the omission of nitrous oxide, and the substitution of remifentanil for fentanyl. In the designated patients, dexamethasone 4 mg or droperidol 1.25 mg intravenous (IV) were administered within 20 minutes after the start of anesthesia, and ondansetron 4 mg IV was administered during the last 20 minutes of surgery. A nonsteroidal anti-inflammatory medication was administered intraoperatively for postoperative pain, and administration of postoperative opioids was left to the discretion of the anesthesiologist. Patients assigned to remifentanil received a weight-based amount of opioid at the end of surgery. Postoperatively, patients requiring antiemetic therapy received 4 mg of ondansetron; if symptoms persisted, 4 mg of dexamethasone and 1.25 mg of droperidol were added.

Follow-Up: 24 hours postoperatively.

Endpoints: Primary outcome: incidence of nausea, emetic episodes (retching or vomiting), or both during the first 24 hours postoperatively. Secondary outcomes: number and time of emetic episodes and a rating for the worst episode based on an 11-point scale (where 0 represented no nausea and 10 the most severe nausea possible) assessed after 2 and 24 hours postoperatively.

RESULTS

- Of the 5,161 patients for whom outcome data were available, 81.5% were women, 81.2% were nonsmokers, 54.5% had a history of PONV, and 78.1% received postoperative opioids.
- Baseline characteristics were similar among patients assigned to each intervention.
- Overall, 1,731 of 5,161 patients (34%) had PONV; nausea occurred in 31% of patients, and vomiting occurred in 14% of patients.
- Among the patients who had symptoms, the median and mean ratings for the maximum nausea level were 5 and 5.7, respectively. The median and mean numbers of emetic episodes were 1 and 1.5, respectively.
- Group-specific PONV rates ranged from 59% (patients receiving volatile anesthesia, nitrous oxide, fentanyl, and no antiemetics) to 17% (patients receiving propofol, remifentanil, ondansetron, dexamethasone, and droperidol).
- There were no significant differences among the antiemetics, any pair of antiemetics, or type of volatile anesthetic (isoflurane, sevoflurane, or desflurane) with regard to the incidence of PONV.
- Each antiemetic reduced the incidence of PONV by approximately 26%, substituting propofol for volatile anesthesia reduced the incidence of PONV by 19%, and use of nitrogen (air) rather than nitrous oxide reduced the incidence of PONV by 12%.
- The use of remifentanil rather than fentanyl did not significantly reduce the incidence of PONV. Remifentanil was associated with increased use of intraoperative vasoconstrictors and postoperative shivering.
- Increasing the number of antiemetics administered reduced the incidence of PONV from 52% when no antiemetics were used to 37%, 28%, and 22% when one, two, and three antiemetics, respectively, were administered, corresponding to a 26% reduction in the relative risk for PONV for each additional antiemetic used.

- Only one significant interaction between treatment and confounding factors was identified: droperidol significantly reduced the risk for PONV among women but not men ($P < 0.001$).
- The relative risk for PONV was similar for all types of surgery with the exception of hysterectomy and possibly cholecystectomy when corrected for major risk factors.

Criticisms and Limitations: Certain elements of intraoperative and post-operative management were left to the discretion of the anesthesiologist and not standardized. This study may not apply to all patients because it does not evaluate the effect of antiemetic strategies in patients with a risk for PONV less than 40%. PONV was treated with the same agents that were used for prophylaxis.

Other Relevant Studies and Information:

- In patients for whom preoperative PONV prophylaxis with ondansetron is not successful, a repeat dose of ondansetron in the postanesthesia care unit does not appear to offer additional control of PONV.[2]
- Duration of exposure to nitrous oxide of less than 1 hour has little effect on the rate of PONV. The risk ratio for PONV increases approximately 20% per hour after the first 45 minutes of exposure to nitrous oxide. This duration-related effect may be due to disturbance of methionine and folate metabolism.[3]
- Severe PONV occurs more frequently with the use of nitrous oxide, but the increased risk is nearly eliminated by antiemetic prophylaxis. Severe PONV is associated with postoperative fever, poor quality of recovery, and prolonged hospitalization.[4]
- The American Society of Anesthesiologists Practice Guidelines for Postanesthetic Care[5] state that "periodic assessment of nausea and vomiting should be performed routinely during emergence and recovery." For the prevention and treatment of nausea and vomiting, antiemetic agents should be used when indicated, and multiple antiemetic agents may be used when indicated.

Summary and Implications: Each of the three antiemetics in this study (ondansetron, dexamethasone, and droperidol) reduced the risk for PONV by approximately 26%; substituting propofol for volatile anesthetic reduced the risk by 19%; and substituting nitrogen (air) for nitrous oxide reduced the risk by 12%. A maximum reduction of 70% in the relative risk for PONV can be expected when total intravenous anesthesia is used with three antiemetics. The appropriate approach to the management of PONV depends on the patient's baseline risk factors as well as the likelihood of adverse events and costs from the antiemetic medications.

CLINICAL CASE: POSTOPERATIVE NAUSEA AND VOMITING PROPHYLAXIS

Case History

A 45-year-old woman presents for laparoscopic cholecystectomy. The patient is a chronic smoker and has a history of motion sickness. Based on the scheduled procedure and the patient's risk factors, describe a possible prophylactic strategy for PONV.

Suggested Answer

The patient has risk factors for PONV (female gender, history of motion sickness, surgical procedure) and should therefore receive PONV prophylaxis. One possible strategy could be to administer dexamethasone 4 mg IV at the induction of anesthesia and ondansetron 4 mg IV 20 minutes before emergence. The use of nitrous oxide should be minimized to less than 1 hour in duration. Propofol could be used for maintenance instead of volatile anesthetics. If the patient develops PONV in the recovery room, treatment with agents other than those used for prophylaxis, such as dimenhydrinate, is advised.

References

1. Apfel CC, Korttila K, Abdalla M, et al. A factorial trial of six interventions for the prevention of postoperative nausea and vomiting. *N Engl J Med.* 2004 Jun 10;350(24):2441–51.
2. Kovac AL, O'Connor TA, Pearman MH, et al. Efficacy of repeat intravenous dosing of ondansetron in controlling postoperative nausea and vomiting: a randomized, double-blind, placebo-controlled multicenter trial. *J Clin Anesth.* 1999 Sep;11(6):453–59.
3. Peyton PJ, Wu CY. Nitrous oxide–related postoperative nausea and vomiting depends on duration of exposure. *Anesthesiology.* 2014 May;120(5):1137–45.

4. Myles PS, Chan MT, Kasza J, et al. Severe PONV, which is seen in more than 10% of patients, is associated with postoperative fever, poor quality of recovery, and prolonged hospitalization. *Anesthesiology.* 2016 May;124(5):1032–40

5. Apfelbaum JL, Silverstein JH, Chung FF, et al. Practice guidelines for postanesthetic care: an updated report by the American Society of Anesthesiologists Task Force on Postanesthetic Care. *Anesthesiology.* 2013 Feb;118(2):291–307.

29

Postoperative Oxygen Desaturation

A Comparison of Regional Anesthesia vs. Continuous Administration of Opioids

These results suggest that postoperative pain relief using regional anaesthesia has a greater margin of safety in terms of respiratory side effects than does the continuous administration of opiates.

—CATLEY ET AL.[1]

Research Question: What are the effects of regional anesthesia vs. continuous administration of opioids on respiratory function following general anesthesia for major surgery?

Year Study Published: 1985.

Study Location: Northwick Park Hospital in Harrow, Middlesex, England.

Who Was Studied: Adult patients undergoing open elective cholecystectomy (using a Kocher's incision) or total hip replacement.

Who Was Excluded: Patients who were smokers, had cardiopulmonary disease, a body mass index (BMI) less than 19 or greater than 25, were American Society of Anesthesiologists (ASA) physical status III or higher, and had baseline respiratory inductive plethysmograph (RIP) examination signals not in phase or room air oxygen saturation below 96%.

How Many Patients: 32.

Study Overview: See Figure 29.1 for an overview of the study's design.

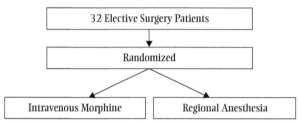

Figure 29.1 Summary of the study design.

Study Intervention: Open cholecystectomy and hip replacement patients were randomized into two groups for analgesia: intravenous morphine and regional anesthesia. All patients received intramuscular opioids 1 hour before surgery. Hip replacement patients randomized to regional anesthesia had a lumbar epidural catheter placed before induction. Intraoperatively, the regional anesthesia group did not receive opiates while the intravenous morphine group received 0.04 mg/kg of morphine on skin closure. Postoperatively, patients in the intravenous morphine group received an infusion of morphine at 1 mg/min until pain was appreciably reduced; the total dose required to achieve adequate analgesia was repeated as a continuous infusion over the subsequent 24 hours (dose was increased if needed). Regional anesthesia patients received bupivacaine injections through the epidural catheter after hip replacement or for T6 to T10 intercostal nerve blocks after cholecystectomy. Pain assessments were obtained every 3-4 hours postoperatively.

Follow-Up: 48 hours postoperatively.

Endpoints: Postoperative pain (measured using a 10-cm linear analog scale and a five-point verbal rating score), episodes of oxygen desaturation, ventilatory pattern disturbances, and sleep stage (Rechtschaffen and Kales[2] scoring criteria).

RESULTS

- The study groups were similar with respect to demographics. There were no significant differences in preoperative oxygen saturation, duration of anesthesia, or mean pain scores between analgesic groups or mean pain scores between surgical groups. Cholecystectomy patients had longer anesthesia times compared with hip replacement patients.

- Morphine infusion rates ranged between 0.25 and 1.95 mg/h, with a mean rate (±SD) of 0.76 ± 0.41 mg/h. After 48 hours postoperatively, all patients reported their analgesia as adequate, but not complete.
- Mean hourly oxygen saturations were obtained by excluding transient oximetry decreases; mean oximetry readings in the morphine group were consistently lower compared with the regional anesthesia group during the 16-hour postoperative observation period. Oxygen saturations in both analgesic groups increased gradually over the 16 hours but did not return to baseline preoperative levels during this time period.
- A total of 456 pronounced desaturation episodes (Sao_2 <80%) lasting between 5 and 120 seconds were recorded in 10 patients during sleep, all of whom were in the morphine analgesic group with no difference between the surgical groups. Nearly all episodes were associated with obstructive apnea or paradoxic breathing.
- There was a significant difference in the lowest oxygen saturations between the morphine and regional anesthesia groups ($P < 0.01$).
- All types of ventilatory disturbance (central apnea, obstructive apnea, paradoxic breathing, slow respiratory rate, and small tidal volume) were more common in patients receiving morphine rather than regional anesthesia. The number of patients with central and obstructive apnea was significantly different in the two analgesic groups ($P = 0.012$ and $P = 0.029$, respectively).
- The incidence of central apnea, slow respiratory rate, and desaturation episodes decreased as the postoperative period progressed.
- The incidence of respiratory disturbances increased with age and was more common in patients in the morphine group who were older than 65 years.
- Electroencephalogram (EEG) arousal and transient hyperventilation were frequently seen before central apnea episodes, which were never associated with desaturation. Obstructive apnea episodes were often preceded by paradoxic breathing with snoring, and EEG arousal was frequently associated with the end of an episode of obstructive apnea.
- Patients in the two analgesic groups had comparable total sleep durations, but the sleep stage was difficult to summarize during ventilatory disturbances.

Criticisms and Limitations: Study patients were generally healthy (nonsmokers, not obese, ASA physical status I or II, and no cardiovascular disease) and were relatively young (the oldest patient was 73 years old). Pain scores were obtained only at rest.

Other Relevant Studies and Information:

- A retrospective, propensity score–matched study examining the benefit of avoiding general anesthesia in patients with chronic obstructive pulmonary disease[3] found that the use of regional anesthesia was associated with lower incidences of composite morbidity, pneumonia, prolonged ventilator dependence, and unplanned postoperative intubation.
- A study examining predictors of desaturation[4] in 502 patients in the immediate postoperative period found significant predictors of desaturation after general anesthesia to included patients' sedation score, low respiratory rate, and transport without oxygen.

Summary and Implications: This study demonstrated that narcotic analgesia is an important cause of oxygen desaturation and ventilatory disturbances during sleep in postoperative patients. The transient nature of desaturations and ventilatory disturbances highlighted the need for continuous monitoring techniques in the postoperative period.

CLINICAL CASE: GENERAL VS. REGIONAL ANESTHESIA

Case History
A 68-year-old woman with a history of chronic obstructive pulmonary disease requiring occasional home oxygen at night presents for total hip replacement. She reports orthopnea and sleeps semi-upright in a recliner or with multiple pillows. Given her history of pulmonary disease, how should this patient be managed to reduce postoperative pulmonary complications?

Suggested Answer
Multimodal analgesia should be used and narcotics minimized in this patient. Regional anesthesia would be preferable for postoperative pain management. Given the history of orthopnea, this patient would likely not be able to tolerate the procedure under a spinal or epidural with sedation. General anesthesia should be focused on minimizing atelectasis and optimizing pulmonary function.

References

1. Catley DM, Thornton C, Jordan C, Lehane JR, Royston D, Jones JG. Pronounced, episodic oxygen desaturation in the postoperative period: its association with ventilatory pattern and analgesic regimen. *Anesthesiology.* 1985 Jul;63(1):20–8.
2. Rechtschaffen A, Kales A (eds): A manual of standardized terminology, techniques and scoring systems for sleep stages in human subjects. Washington DC: Public Health Service, US Government Printing Office, 1968.
3. Hausman MS Jr, Jewell ES, Engoren M. Regional versus general anesthesia in surgical patients with chronic obstructive pulmonary disease: does avoiding general anesthesia reduce the risk of postoperative complications? *Anesth Analg.* 2015 Jun;120(6):1405–12.
4. Siddiqui N, Arzola C, Teresi J, Fox G, Guerina L, Friedman Z. Predictors of desaturation in the postoperative anesthesia care unit: an observational study. *J Clin Anesth.* 2013 Dec;25(8):612–7.

30

Surgical Site Infections Following Ambulatory Surgery Procedures

Among patients undergoing ambulatory surgery, rates of postsurgical visits for clinically significant surgical site infections were low relative to all causes; however, they may represent a substantial number of adverse outcomes in aggregate.

—OWENS ET AL.[1]

Research Question: What is the incidence of clinically significant surgical site infections (CS-SSIs) following low- to moderate-risk ambulatory surgery in patients at low risk for surgical complications?

Funding: Agency for Healthcare Research and Quality.

Year Study Began: 2010.

Year Study Published: 2014.

Study Location: California, Florida, Georgia, Hawaii, Missouri, Nebraska, New York, and Tennessee.

Who Was Studied: Encounter data for patients who underwent one of 12 selected low- to moderate-risk ambulatory surgical procedures covering a range of specialties—general surgery, orthopedics, neurosurgery, gynecology, and urology. Selected procedures included laparoscopic cholecystectomy, six types of hernia repair (open and laparoscopic for inguinal or femoral, umbilical, and incisional or abdominal), spinal laminectomy or diskectomy, anterior cruciate ligament (ACL) repair, vaginal and abdominal hysterectomy, and transurethral prostatectomy.

Who Was Excluded: Patients who experienced hospital events (inpatient or ambulatory center) in the 30 days before surgery; were <18 years of age; were not discharged to home; underwent more than one surgery on the same day; had an infection coded on the same day as the surgery; had a length of stay ≥2 days or were admitted in December or January; underwent surgery for the treatment of cancer.

How Many Patients: 284,098.

Study Overview: See Figure 30.1 for an overview of the study's design.

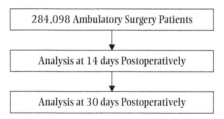

Figure 30.1 Summary of the study design.

Study Intervention: Encounter data were abstracted from the Agency for Healthcare Research and Quality Healthcare Cost and Utilization Project State Ambulatory Surgery Databases and State Inpatient Databases from eight states in 2010. These data were analyzed to identify postsurgical encounters for CS-SSIs that required a postsurgical acute care visit (subsequent hospitalization or ambulatory surgical visit for infection). CS-SSI cases were identified using *ICD-9-CM* diagnosis codes, *ICD-9-CM* procedures or *CPT* procedures, or both. A sensitivity analysis was conducted to determine the validity of the algorithm. Rates of ambulatory surgical visits or postsurgical inpatient stays for all causes were computed to indicate the relative importance of SSIs as a reason for postsurgical visits.

Follow-Up: 14 and 30 days postoperatively.

Endpoints: Primary outcome: rate of postsurgical acute care visits following each of the selected surgical procedures. Secondary outcomes: time between the index ambulatory surgical procedure and a subsequent ambulatory surgical visit or inpatient stay; rate of ambulatory surgical visits or postsurgical inpatient stays for all causes.

RESULTS

- The overall rate of postsurgical visits for all causes (e.g., CS-SSIs, postoperative pain and swelling, gastrointestinal, respiratory) was 19.99 per 1,000 ambulatory surgical procedures within 14 days and 33.62 per 1,000 ambulatory surgical procedures within 30 days postoperatively.
- The rate of postsurgical acute care visits for CS-SSIs within 14 days of surgery was 3.09 per 1,000 ambulatory surgical procedures. When follow-up was extended to 30 days postoperatively, the rate of postsurgical acute care visits for CS-SSIs rose to 4.84 per 1,000 ambulatory surgical procedures.
- The visit rates varied by type of ambulatory surgery, and at 14 days postoperatively they ranged from 0.27 per 1,000 repairs of inguinal or femoral hernia to 6.44 per 1,000 vaginal hysterectomies.
- Approximately two-thirds (63.7%) of all postsurgical visits for CS-SSIs occurred within 14 days of ambulatory surgery. This pattern was similar for each type of surgery except laparoscopic repair of inguinal or femoral hernia, open repair of incisional or abdominal hernia, and spine surgery; less than half of the postsurgical visits for CS-SSIs for these procedures occurred in the first 14 days.
- There was no significant difference in postsurgical visits for CS-SSIs following open vs. laparoscopic repair, except for repair of inguinal or femoral hernia.
- Approximately 90% of postsurgical acute care visits for CS-SSIs were treated in the inpatient setting.

Criticisms and Limitations: This study analyzed patient data for eight states, which represented approximately one third of the population in the United States; results may not reflect CS-SSI rates in specific areas of the country. The data did not capture visits to nonhospital facilities such as physician offices and the emergency department, thereby excluding CS-SSIs that were managed in the outpatient setting.

Other Relevant Studies and Information:

- The cost associated with surgical site infections is substantial. The Veterans Health Administration calculated that if hospitals in the 10th percentile for SSI rates (i.e., the worst hospitals) reduced their SSI rates to the rates of hospitals in the 50th percentile, savings would total approximately $6.7 million per year.[2]
- Smoking is a modifiable risk factor for the development of surgical site infection because postoperative healing complications occur significantly more often in smokers compared with nonsmokers and in former smokers compared with patients who never smoked.[3]

Summary and Implications: This retrospective analysis found that the overall rate of CS-SSIs following ambulatory surgery is relatively low, at approximately 3.09 per 1,000 ambulatory surgical procedures. However, because of the high volume of ambulatory cases annually, the actual number of acute care visits due to CS-SSIs is large in aggregate. More than 90% of the CS-SSIs in this analysis required treatment in an inpatient setting, demonstrating a substantial cost burden. Thus, surgical site infections merit quality improvement efforts to minimize their occurrence.

CLINICAL CASE: SURGICAL SITE INFECTION

Case History

A 57-year-old man presents for a preoperative evaluation before his upcoming elective ventral hernia repair in 8 weeks. The patient currently smokes cigarettes daily. During the interview, he expresses concern for developing a surgical site infection, which occurred following his laparoscopic cholecystectomy several years prior. How should his tobacco use be addressed?

Suggested Answer

The patient should be counseled on smoking cessation. The direct impact of smoking on outcomes such as surgical site infection should be discussed. Resources for smoking cessation should be provided.

References

1. Owens PL, Barrett ML, Raetzman S, Maggard-Gibbons M, Steiner CA. Surgical site infections following ambulatory surgery procedures. *JAMA*. 2014 Feb 19;311(7):709–16.
2. Schweizer ML, Cullen JJ, Perencevich EN, Vaughan Sarrazin MS. Costs associated with surgical site infections in veterans affairs hospitals. *JAMA Surg*. 2014 Jun;149(6):575–81.
3. Sorensen LT. Wound healing and infection in surgery. The clinical impact of smoking and smoking cessation: a systematic review and meta-analysis. *Arch Surg*. 2012 Apr;147(4):373–83.

31

Care Coordination

The [Project] RED intervention decreased hospital utilization (combined emergency department visits and readmissions) within 30 days of discharge by about 30% among patients on a general medicine service of an urban, academic medical center.

—JACK ET AL.[1]

Research Question: Is it possible to reduce the rate of repeat emergency department and hospital visits after discharge by improving care coordination?[1]

Funding: The Agency for Healthcare Research and Quality and the National Heart, Lung, and Blood Institute, National Institutes of Health.

Year Study Began: 2004.

Year Study Published: 2009.

Study Location: Boston Medical Center, Boston, Massachusetts.

Who Was Studied: Adults admitted to the general medicine service of an urban, academic medical center that serves an "ethnically diverse patient population."

Who Was Excluded: Patients without a home telephone, those unable to "comprehend study details and the consent process in English," those on a suicide watch, and those who were blind or deaf. In addition, patients were excluded if they were not discharged home (e.g., if they were discharged to a nursing facility).

How Many Patients: 749.

Study Overview: See Figure 31.1 for an overview of the study's design.

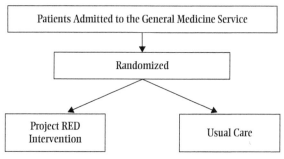

Figure 31.1 Summary of the trial design.

Study Intervention: Patients in the Project RED (Reengineered Discharge) group were assigned to nurse discharge advocates who provided the patients with the following services and assistance during the hospitalization:

- Education about their condition
- Assistance with postdischarge appointment scheduling and planning
- Education about medications and medication reconciliation on discharge
- Education about how to address postdischarge problems (e.g., whom to contact)

At the time of discharge, the advocates gave each patient a written discharge plan listing the reason for hospitalization, the discharge medication list, contact information for the patient's ambulatory care providers, and information about postdischarge appointments and testing. The discharge advocates transmitted the postdischarge care plan and the hospital discharge summary to each patient's ambulatory providers.

Two to four days after discharge, a clinical pharmacist called each patient "to reinforce the discharge plan, review medications, and solve problems."

Patients in the control group received usual hospital and postdischarge care.

Follow-Up: 30 days.

Endpoints: Primary outcome: emergency department and hospital visits within 30 days of hospital discharge. Secondary outcomes: patients' knowledge about their discharge diagnoses; the percentage of patients visiting their primary care doctors after discharge; and "self-reported preparedness for discharge."

RESULTS

- Among patients in the Project RED group, 83% were discharged with a written discharge plan and 91% had their discharge information transmitted to their primary care doctors within 24 hours of discharge.
- After discharge, pharmacists were able to reach 62% of patients in the Project RED group by telephone, and more than half of the patients who were contacted had medication problems requiring "corrective action."
- Project RED discharge advocates spent an estimated 87.5 minutes per patient, while pharmacists spent an estimated 26 minutes per patient.
- There were fewer emergency department and hospital visits after discharge in the Project RED group vs. the control group (Table 31.1).
- Project RED was most effective in preventing emergency department and hospital visits among patients with the highest hospital utilization during the previous 6 months.
- Overall, Project RED lowered health care costs by an average of $412 per patient (mainly by preventing emergency department and hospital visits); the authors did not indicate whether these savings offset the program costs, however.

Table 31.1. SUMMARY OF THE TRIAL'S KEY FINDINGS

Outcome	Control Group	Project RED Group	P Value
Total hospital and emergency department visits after discharge	0.451*	0.314*	0.009
Emergency department visits	0.245*	0.165*	0.014
Hospital visits	0.207*	0.149*	0.090
Patients able to identify their discharge diagnoses	70%	79%	0.017
Patients visiting their primary doctors after discharge	44%	62%	<0.001
Patients reporting that they felt prepared for discharge	55%	65%	0.013

*Mean number of visits per patient per month.

Criticisms and Limitations: Because of staffing limitations, the nurse discharge advocates were only able to enroll two to three patients per day and did not enroll any patients on some weekends and holidays.

Because Project RED involved multiple components (i.e., education in the hospital, postdischarge planning, and postdischarge outreach), it is not clear which component of the program was responsible for its success.

The Project RED intervention might not have been as effective in other health care settings. For example, patients of higher socioeconomic status might not require as much assistance with postdischarge planning.

Other Relevant Studies and Information:

- Other studies have also demonstrated that care coordination programs at the time of hospital discharge can reduce the rate of repeat emergency department and hospital visits[2,3]; not all such programs have been successful, however.[4-6]

Summary and Implications: The Project RED program substantially reduced repeat emergency department and hospital visits by improving care coordination at the time of hospital discharge.

CLINICAL CASE: CARE COORDINATION AT HOSPITAL DISCHARGE

Case History
A community hospital wants to improve care coordination for its patients at the time of discharge. What are the challenges to implementing a program like Project RED?

Suggested Answer
Perhaps the largest obstacle to implementing a program like Project RED is financial because it is not clear where the funding for such a program should come from. Improving care coordination does not generate revenue for the hospital (in fact, it could have the opposite effect by reducing emergency department and hospital visits). Moreover, insurance companies do not typically reimburse for programs like Project RED.

The Medicare program is currently trying to restructure financial incentives to promote programs like Project RED that improve health care quality and efficiency. For example, Medicare is beginning to penalize hospitals with high readmission rates in an attempt to promote care coordination at discharge.

References

1. Jack BW, Chetty VK, Anthony D, et al. A reengineered hospital discharge program to decrease rehospitalization. *Ann Intern Med.* 2009;150:178–87.
2. Coleman EA, Parry C, Chalmers S, et al. The care transitions intervention: results of a random controlled trial. *Arch Intern Med.* 2006;166:1822–28.
3. Naylor MD, Brooten D, Campbell R, et al. Comprehensive discharge planning and home follow-up of hospitalized elders: a randomized clinical trial. *JAMA.* 1999;281:613–20.
4. Weinberger M, Oddone EZ, Henderson WG. Does increased access to primary care reduce hospital readmissions? Veterans Affairs Cooperative Study Group on Primary Care and Hospital Readmission. *N Engl J Med.* 1996;334:1441–47.
5. Shepperd S, Parkes J, McClaren J, Phillips C. Discharge planning from hospital to home. *Cochrane Database Syst Rev.* 2004:CD000313.
6. Hesselink G, Schoonhoven L, Barach P, et al. Improving patient handovers from hospital to primary care: a systematic review. *Ann Intern Med.* 2012;157(6):417.

32

Pulmonary Aspiration

Clinical Significance in the Perioperative Period

This study suggests that patients with clinically apparent aspiration who do not develop symptoms within 2 h are unlikely to have respiratory sequelae.

—WARNER ET AL.[1]

Research Question: What is the incidence and clinical significance of pulmonary aspiration during the perioperative period based on the predictive potential of common clinical findings?

Funding: Mayo Foundation and the Anesthesia Patient Safety Foundation.

Year Study Began: 1985.

Year Study Published: 1993.

Study Location: Mayo Clinic, Rochester, Minnesota.

Who Was Studied: Perioperative records for patients 18 years or older who underwent 215,488 consecutive general anesthetics for elective or emergent procedures at a single institution during a 6-year period.

How Many Patients: 172,335.

Study Overview: See Figure 32.1 for an overview of the study's design.

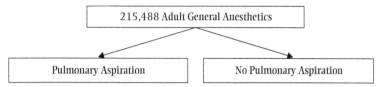

Figure 32.1 Summary of the study design.

Study Intervention: This study used an integrated database of patient records to determine the incidence of pulmonary aspiration in the intraoperative and immediate postoperative periods. This database was reviewed monthly, and providers were interviewed about the specifics of each aspiration occurrence. Pulmonary aspiration was defined as "presence of bilious secretions or particulate matter in the tracheobronchial tree or, in patients who did not have their tracheobronchial airways directly examined after regurgitation, a postoperative chest roentgenogram with infiltrates not identified by preoperative roentgenogram or physical examination." Additional databases (master billing records, medical diagnoses, laboratory investigations, and radiologic interpretations) were used to identify cases requiring intensive care and respiratory services with the diagnosis of pulmonary aspiration, adult respiratory distress syndrome, pneumonia, or pneumonitis. Following a pulmonary aspiration event, findings elicited included the development of a new cough or wheeze, hemoglobin oxygen saturation on room air of ≥10% less than the preoperative value, alveolar-arterial oxygen tension ≥300 mm Hg in patients who remained intubated, and radiographic abnormalities within 2 hours of aspiration or the completion of anesthetic.

Follow-Up: Patients were initially assessed 2 hours postoperatively. Data on patient disposition, use of intensive care, ventilatory support, and pulmonary outcomes were collected from administrative records.

Endpoints: Clinical significance and the predictive potential of common clinical findings after perioperative pulmonary aspiration.

RESULTS

- There were 172,335 adult patients who underwent 215,488 general anesthetics, of which 13,427 were for emergency procedures.
- Pulmonary aspiration occurred in 67 cases (1:3,216 anesthetics). The overall mortality rate from pulmonary aspiration was 1:71,829 anesthetics.

- Both increasing American Society of Anesthesiologists (ASA) physical status and emergency procedures were associated with a greater risk for pulmonary aspiration.
- The following were not found to be independent risk factors for pulmonary aspiration: age, gender, pregnancy, ingestion of a meal within 3 hours, concurrent opioid administration, body mass index ≥35, individual comorbid diseases, experience and type of anesthesia provider, type of surgical procedure.
- Most aspiration events occurred during laryngoscopy (32.9%) and extubation (35.9%).
- Of the 52 patients who experienced pulmonary aspiration while undergoing elective procedures, 24 had predisposing conditions; all 15 patients who experienced pulmonary aspiration while undergoing emergency procedures had predisposing conditions.
- Of the patients who aspirated and had predisposing conditions to pulmonary aspiration, 18 received one or more of preoperative oral antacids, oral or parenteral histamine-2 receptor antagonists, or medications that improve gastric emptying; pulmonary complications developed in approximately equal percentages between those patients who received and did not receive acid aspiration prophylaxis.
- The most common predisposing condition in all cases of pulmonary aspiration was gastrointestinal obstruction (21 patients). Other predisposing conditions included lack of coordination of swallowing (6 patients), depressed level of consciousness (6 patients), previous esophageal surgery (3 patients), and recent meal (3 patients).
- Of the 67 pulmonary aspiration events, 1 patient did not survive the procedure because of bleeding, 42 patients did not develop signs or symptoms within 2 hours of the aspiration or completion of anesthetic (and none required intensive care or respiratory support or developed pulmonary complications), and the remaining 24 patients developed one or more signs or symptoms of aspiration—cough or wheeze (10 patients), a decrease in oxygen saturation ≥10% less from preoperative value (10 patients), alveolar-arterial oxygen tension ≥300 mm Hg (1 patient), and radiologic evidence of pulmonary aspiration within 2 hours of aspiration or completion of anesthetic (12 patients).
- Of the 24 patients who developed one or more signs or symptoms of aspiration, 18 required intensive care or respiratory support or developed pulmonary complications, and of these, 13 required

postoperative mechanical ventilatory support for >6 hours, seven for <24 hours, and six for ≥24 hours.

- All six patients who required mechanical ventilation for ≥24 hours developed adult respiratory distress syndrome; three of these patients died of respiratory failure.
- Pneumonia with an identifiable source (*Klebsiella*) developed in only one patient.
- None of the patients received steroids or antibiotics for prophylaxis.

Criticisms and Limitations: The authors of the study state that underreporting of the incidence of aspiration was possible but not probable given that multiple databases were queried and validity checks did not identify additional cases that were not already obtained from the database searches. As much as 1 month may have passed between the time of the aspiration event to when providers were interviewed, raising the possibility of recall bias.

Other Relevant Studies and Information:

- One recent study reviewed pulmonary aspiration in perioperative medicine and concluded that any patient with symptoms following an aspiration that last for more than 2 hours in the recovery room should be admitted to an intensive care unit for observation.[2]
- Airway pepsin has been used as a biomarker for gastric-to-pulmonary aspiration. Bohman et al.[3] demonstrated that enzymatically active pepsin C, but not gastric-specific pepsin A, is frequently detected in the lower airways of patients following endotracheal intubation who otherwise have no risk factors for aspiration. Nonspecific pepsin assays should therefore be used and interpreted with caution as a biomarker of gastropulmonary aspiration.
- Anesthesia impairs the coordination between swallowing and respiration. Mild hypercapnia increases the frequency of swallowing during anesthesia and the likelihood of pathologic swallowing; the risk for aspiration may be increased when ventilator drive is stimulated during anesthesia.[4]
- In older adults without symptoms, pharyngeal function is often impaired. Any residual effect of a neuromuscular-blocking agent after general anesthesia may worsen this age-associated impairment of

pharyngeal function and is a possible cause of postoperative aspiration in the older adult surgical population.[5]

Summary and Implications: This study showed that pulmonary aspiration among surgical patients was associated with increasing ASA physical status and emergency procedures. Patient with clinically apparent pulmonary aspiration who do not develop signs or symptoms within 2 hours in the immediate postoperative period are unlikely to have respiratory sequelae.

CLINICAL CASE: PULMONARY ASPIRATION

Case History

A 47-year-old woman underwent urgent exploratory laparoscopy and lysis of adhesions for a small bowel obstruction. During the procedure, a nasogastric tube was placed for decompression and maintained on low continuous suction. At the end of the procedure, on extubation, the patient vomited a small amount of nonparticulate, bilious gastric content. The oral pharynx was immediately suctioned. The patient experienced a brief episode of laryngospasm followed by coughing. Given the possible aspiration event, how should the patient be managed postoperatively?

Suggested Answer

The patient should be examined and closely monitored from a respiratory standpoint during the initial recovery period. Findings such as wheezing on physical examination, the development of a cough, or a significant decrease in oxygen saturation from baseline should prompt radiographic studies and transfer of the patient to a monitored setting.

References

1. Warner MA, Warner ME, Weber JG. Clinical significance of pulmonary aspiration during the perioperative period. *Anesthesiology.* 1993 Jan;78(1):56–62.
2. Abdulla S. Pulmonary aspiration in perioperative medicine. *Acta Anaesthesiol Belg.* 2013;64(1):1–13.
3. Bohman JK, Kor DJ, Kashyap R, et al. Airway pepsin levels in otherwise healthy surgical patients receiving general anesthesia with endotracheal intubation. *Chest.* 2013 May;143(5):1407–13.

4. D'Angelo OM, Diaz-Gil D, Nunn D, et al. Anesthesia and increased hypercarbic drive impair the coordination between breathing and swallowing. *Anesthesiology.* 2014 Dec;121(6):1175–83.

5. Asai T, Isono S. Residual neuromuscular blockade after anesthesia: a possible cause of postoperative aspiration-induced pneumonia. *Anesthesiology.* 2014 Feb;120(2):260–2.

33

Postoperative Pain Experience

Our findings suggest that greater awareness of the importance of managing pain and the dedication of resources to pain control are needed to improve postoperative pain management.

—APFELBAUM ET AL.[1]

Research Question: What is the postoperative pain experience in the United States, and what is the level of patient satisfaction with pain medications, success of patient education, and patient perceptions about postoperative pain and pain medications?

Funding: Pharmacia, Inc.

Year Study Published: 2003.

Study Location: Randomly selected households throughout the United States.

Who Was Studied: Adults who had surgery within the past 5 years.

Who Was Excluded: Adults who had not had surgery within the past 5 years.

How Many Patients: 250.

Study Overview: See Figure 33.1 for an overview of the study's design.

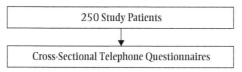

Figure 33.1 Summary of the study design.

Study Intervention: The list of potential study subjects was obtained from National Family Opinion–WorldGroup, a market research organization. The initial panel of households was randomly selected to be representative of the US population in terms of geography, age of household head, household income and size, and market size. A random sample of 666 adults were contacted to obtain 250 eligible participants. Interviews were conducted by telephone with predetermined questions regarding the pain experience.

Follow-Up: This was a cross-sectional study.

Endpoints: Questions on the survey addressed the presence and severity of postoperative pain, pain medications received, adverse effects of pain medications, satisfaction with pain medications after surgery (both while in the hospital and 2 weeks after discharge), and other factors.

RESULTS:

- The majority of patients were women (65%) with a mean age of 46 years.
- Type of facility: 52% of patients underwent inpatient surgery, 38% had outpatient surgery, and the remaining 10% underwent procedures in a doctor's office, outpatient clinic, or freestanding surgery center.
- Length of time since surgery: 60% of outpatient procedures had occurred within 1 year of the survey, and 5% had occurred between 4 and 5 years prior. For inpatient procedures, 40% occurred within 1 year of the survey, and 23% had occurred between 4 and 5 years prior.
- Patients were most concerned about pain after surgery (59%) and whether the surgery would improve their condition (51%). Other concerns included recovery and whether or not health care professionals would be responsive and sensitive to their medical needs.
- Overall, 82% of patients reported experiencing pain from the time of surgery until 2 weeks after discharge. Of these patients, 47% experienced moderate pain and 39% experienced severe to extreme pain.

- Postoperative pain appeared to be better controlled before discharge: 58% of patients experienced pain before discharge compared with 75% after discharge.
- Overall, 82% of patients received pain medication in the inpatient or outpatient setting. After discharge, 76% of patients received pain medications. Of these patients, almost 90% were satisfied with their pain medication.
- Two-thirds of patients reported a preoperative discussion with a health care professional regarding postoperative pain management. Postoperatively, two-thirds of patient reported being asked by a health care professional about their pain. Preoperative and postoperative discussions about pain were most frequently performed by a nurse.
- Nearly all (94%) patients believed pain medication caused adverse effects, and 72% of patients reported that they would choose a nonnarcotic drug (main reasons being less addictive properties and fewer adverse effects). Most commonly reported adverse effects were drowsiness, nausea, and constipation.

Criticisms and Limitations: This was a retrospective survey that is subject to recall bias. The study included only 250 patients.

Other Relevant Studies and Information:

- Acute postoperative pain can progress to persistent postsurgical pain in a significant percentage of patients.[2]
- A recently published combined systematic review and meta-analysis demonstrated that perioperative administration of gabapentin and pregabalin are effective in reducing the incidence of chronic postsurgical pain.[3]

Summary and Implications: The results of this study indicate that most patients experience moderate to severe pain postoperatively. Additional efforts are required to improve patients' postoperative pain experience.

CLINICAL CASE: POSTOPERATIVE PAIN

Case History

A 52-year-old woman presents for outpatient laparoscopic inguinal hernia repair under general anesthesia. She is otherwise healthy but expresses concerns about postoperative pain management, especially since prior experience with narcotics caused nausea. She is a nonsmoker and reports a history of motion sickness.

Suggested Answer

The patient has multiple risk factors for postoperative nausea and vomiting (PONV), including female gender, nonsmoker, and history of motion sickness, and should therefore receive PONV prophylaxis, especially given a history of nausea with narcotics. If there are no surgical contraindications, ketorolac could be administered for postoperative pain. Additionally, the patient could be premedicated with acetaminophen and gabapentin or pregabalin before induction. A discussion of the plan for postoperative pain management with the patient should occur before the procedure.

References

1. Apfelbaum JL, Chen C, Mehta SS, Gan TJ. Postoperative pain experience: results from a national survey suggest postoperative pain continues to be undermanaged. *Anesth Analg.* 2003 Aug;97(2):534–40, table of contents.
2. Kehlet H, Jensen TS, Woolf CJ. Persistent postsurgical pain: risk factors and prevention. *Lancet.* 2006 May 13;367(9522):1618–25.
3. Clarke H, Bonin RP, Orser BA, Englesakis M, Wijeysundera DN, Katz J. The prevention of chronic postsurgical pain using gabapentin and pregabalin: a combined systematic review and meta-analysis. *Anesth Analg.* 2012 Aug;115(2):428–42.

Pain Anesthesiology

34

An fMRI-Based Neurologic Signature of Physical Pain

We identified an fMRI-based neurologic signature [that is] associated with thermal pain, discriminates physical pain from several other salient, aversive events, and is sensitive to the analgesic effects of opioids.

—WAGER ET AL.[1]

Research Question: Can functional magnetic resonance imaging (fMRI) be used to identify sensitive and specific brain measures of experimental thermal pain in healthy volunteers?

Funding: National Institute on Drug Abuse, National Institute of Mental Health, and National Science Foundation.

Year Study Began: The four individual studies began between 2005 and 2010.

Year Study Published: 2013.

Study Location: Columbia University.

Who Was Studied: Healthy, right-handed adults without a history of psychiatric, neurologic, or pain disorders. Additionally, Study 3 participants experienced an unwanted romantic relationship breakup within 6 months and indicated that thinking about their breakup experience led them to feel rejected.

How Many Patients: 114.

Study Overview: See Figure 34.1 for an overview of the study's design.

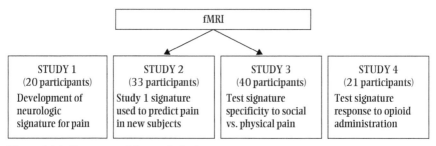

Figure 34.1 Summary of the study design.

Study Intervention: Thermal stimulation was delivered to the volar surface of the left (nondominant) forearm of each subject during fMRI scanning. In Study 1, trials of four intensities were calibrated for each person (warmth and three levels of painful heat) and administered with a warning cue, anticipation period, stimulation period, and pain-recall and rating period. A machine-learning regression technique was used to predict pain reports from the fMRI activity. In Study 2, the neurologic signature identified in Study 1 was tested when participants underwent trials across six temperatures in 1° C increments and after each trial judged whether the stimulus was warm or painful. In Study 3, participants received a painful heat stimulus and a warm stimulus near the pain threshold calibrated for each person. Additionally, Study 3 participants viewed images of their ex-partner and close friend to test signature specificity to social pain vs. physical pain. In Study 4, participants received two administrations of remifentanil infusions during fMRI scanning in two series of trials—an open-infusion series in which participants were aware that they received remifentanil; and a hidden-infusion series in which participants were told that no drug was delivered even through it was administered (remifentanil dosages were individually calibrated to elicit analgesia without sedation).

Endpoints: In Study 1, innocuous warmth was defined as level 1, and three levels of painful heat were defined as levels 3, 5, and 7 on a 9-point visual analog scale (VAS). In Study 2, nonpainful warmth and pain intensity were judged on a 100-point VAS.

RESULTS

- The fMRI neurologic signature included multiple regions of the brain, consistent with the view of pain as a distributed process.
- In Study 1, the fMRI neurologic signature showed sensitivity and specificity of 94% or more in discriminating painful heat from nonpainful warmth, pain anticipation, and pain recall. Forced-choice tests showed 100% sensitivity and specificity for all three comparisons.
- In Study 2, the fMRI neurologic signature derived from Study 1 discriminated between painful heat and nonpainful warmth with 93% sensitivity and specificity. Additionally, the signature response increased monotonically across the six temperatures and correlated with both the reported level of pain and the stimulus temperature.
- In Study 3, the fMRI neurologic signature discriminated between physical and social pain with 85% sensitivity and 73% specificity, as well as with 95% sensitivity and specificity in a forced-choice test of which two conditions was more painful.
- In Study 4, the strength of the fMRI neurologic signature response was substantially reduced when remifentanil was administered.

Criticisms and Limitations: This study was conducted in healthy volunteers without a history of psychiatric, neurologic, or pain disorders; pain classification may be less accurate in patients than in healthy study subjects and may differ according to body site, type of pain (e.g., visceral vs. cutaneous), and clinical cause, necessitating the development of multiple pain signatures. Clinical use of fMRI-based signatures for pain would require calibration across persons, scanning protocols, and research sites.

Other Relevant Studies and Information:

- An fMRI study published in 2014 characterized brain responses to nonnociceptive sensory stimulation in fibromyalgia patients and matched controls. On fMRI, fibromyalgia patients showed strong attenuation of brain responses to nonpainful events in early sensory cortices, accompanied by an amplified response at later stages of sensory integration in the insula. Reduced responses in visual and auditory areas were correlated with subjective sensory hypersensitivity and clinical severity measures.[2]

- An fMRI study published in 2017 identified a brain-based fibromyalgia signature using 37 fibromyalgia patients and 35 matched controls. Combined activity in the neurologic pain signature, fibromyalgia pain, and multisensory patterns classified patients vs. controls with 92% sensitivity and 94% specificity in out-of-sample individuals.[3]

Summary and Implications: This fMRI study identified an interpretable and reproducible neurologic signature of cutaneous pain elicited by noxious heat in healthy volunteers. The interpretation of fMRI neurologic signatures could be useful in situations in which patients are unable to communicate the perception of pain effectively. Further studies are needed to assess whether this signature predicts clinical pain.

References

1. Wager TD, Atlas LY, Lindquist MA, Roy M, Woo CW, Kross E. An fMRI-based neurologic signature of physical pain. *N Engl J Med.* 2013 Apr 11;368(15):1388–97.
2. López-Solà M, Pujol J, Wager TD, et al. Altered functional magnetic resonance imaging responses to nonpainful sensory stimulation in fibromyalgia patients. *Arthritis Rheumatol.* 2014 Nov;66(11):3200–9.
3. López-Solà M, Woo CW, Pujol J, et al. Towards a neurophysiological signature for fibromyalgia. Pain. 2017 Jan;158(1):34–47.

35

Clinical Importance of Changes on a Numerical Pain Rating Scale

> On average, a reduction of approximately two points or a reduction of approximately 30% in the [0-to-10 pain intensity numerical rating scale] represented a clinically important difference.
>
> —Farrar et al.[1]

Research Question: What degree of change on a 0-to-10 pain intensity numerical rating scale (PI-NRS) used for the assessment of chronic pain is associated with clinically important improvement?

Year Study Published: 2001.

Study Location: University of Pennsylvania School of Medicine and Pfizer Global Research and Development.

Who Was Studied: Patient data from 10 completed studies of pregabalin treatment for chronic pain in diabetic neuropathy, postherpetic neuralgia, low back pain, fibromyalgia, and osteoarthritis.

Who Was Excluded: Patients who did not have scores recorded for baseline pain intensity, endpoint pain intensity, or patient global impression of change (PGIC).

How Many Patients: 2,724.

Study Overview: See Figure 35.1 for an overview of the study's design.

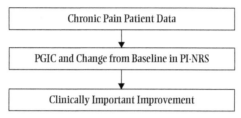

Figure 35.1 Summary of the study design.

Study Intervention: All 10 of the double-blind, placebo-controlled, parallel, multicenter chronic pain studies used a common study design with identical pain measures. Throughout each study of 5 to 12 weeks' duration, patients assessed chronic pain daily using an 11-point PI-NRS, where 0 = no pain and 10 = worst possible pain. The baseline score was the mean of pain scores taken over 7 days before taking study medication. The endpoint score was the mean of the last seven daily scores while receiving study medication. At the endpoint of each study, patients completed the PGIC, and physicians completed a clinical global impression of change (CGIC). The a priori definition of clinical importance included PGIC categories of "much improved" or "very much improved." The change in PI-NRS from baseline was determined as a raw change score and percentage change, and patients were stratified into PGIC categories.

Endpoints: Change from baseline on an 11-point PI-NRS and on a 7-point categorical PGIC scale (very much improved, much improved, minimally improved, no change, minimally worse, much worse, and very much worse).

RESULTS

- On average, among these 10 studies, a decrease of two or more units from baseline in PI-NRS was associated with a PGIC category of "much improved" and a decrease of a least four PI-NRS units was associated with a PGIC category of "very much improved". This change corresponds to percentage changes in PI-NRS of 30% and 50%, respectively.
- The association between PI-NRS and PGIC was consistent across studies regardless of disease model, trial duration, patient demographics

(age, gender), or whether or not the drug was shown to be effective in a particular trial.

- Placebo and active treatment groups had identical changes in PI-NRS associated with each level of PGIC.
- When stratified by baseline pain, higher baseline pain necessitated larger change scores from baseline but similar percentage change to achieve the same level of PGIC.
- Receiver operating characteristics analysis demonstrated a PI-NRS score decrease of 1.74 and a percentage change of 27.9% to be best associated with the a priori definition of clinically important improvement.
- There was a high correlation between the CGIC and the PGIC.

Criticisms and Limitations: Although several disease states were represented in this analysis, the results may not generalize to all chronic pain syndromes, nor to studies with observation periods longer than 12 weeks.

OTHER RELEVANT STUDIES AND INFORMATION:

- The 0-to-10 numerical rating scale is a standard instrument in pain assessment and pain studies. Another commonly used assessment is the 0- to 100-mm visual analog scale (VAS).[2] The VAS is generally completed by patients themselves by placing a mark on a continuous line. The VAS score is determined by measuring in millimeters from the left end of the line to the point that the patient marks.

Summary and Implications: These findings suggest that a PI-NRS score decrease of 1.74 and a percentage change of 27.9% correlate with a clinically important improvement in pain symptoms.

CLINICAL CASE: CHRONIC PAIN MANAGEMENT

Case History

A 46-year-old man with chronic back pain presents for a follow-up appointment. Three months prior, the patient reported a baseline pain score of 7 out of 10. Since his last appointment, the patient has initiated physical therapy and cognitive behavioral therapy and has managed flareups with courses of nonsteroidal anti-inflammatory drugs. The patient is opposed to narcotic medications because of a personal history of narcotic abuse. He states his pain is "much improved" but still rates his average daily back pain a 4 out of 10 in intensity. How should the discrepancy between the residual pain score and the patient's perception of improvement be interpreted?

Suggested Answer
Given that the patient's average pain score improved by 3 points on the 0-to-10 numerical rating scale, this constitutes a clinically important difference.

References

1. Farrar JT, Young JP Jr, LaMoreaux L, Werth JL, Poole RM. Clinical importance of changes in chronic pain intensity measured on an 11-point numerical pain rating scale. *Pain.* 2001 Nov;94(2):149–58.
2. Freud M: The graphic rating scale. J Educ Psychol. 1923 14:83–102.

36

Postinjury Pain Hypersensitivity and NMDA Receptor Antagonists

These results indicate that NMDA receptors are involved in the induction and maintenance of the central sensitization produced by high threshold primary afferent inputs. Because central sensitization is likely to contribute to the post-injury pain hypersensitivity states in man, these data have a bearing both on the potential role of NMDA antagonists for pre-emptive analgesia and for treating established pain states.

—WOOLF AND THOMPSON[1]

Research Question: Are primary afferent-induced hypersensitivity states dependent on the activation of *N*-methyl-D-aspartate (NMDA) receptors, and is windup (perceived increase in pain intensity with a repeatedly delivered stimulus) a possible trigger for the production of central hypersensitivity?

Funding: Medical Research Council and Welcome Trust.

Year Study Published: 1991.

Study Location: University College London, London, England.

Who Was Studied: Adult Sprague-Dawley rats.

Study Overview: See Figure 36.1 for an overview of the study's design.

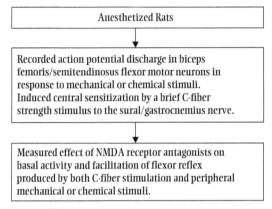

Figure 36.1 Summary of the study design.

Study Intervention: Study animals were anesthetized, paralyzed, and artificially ventilated, and their rectal temperature, expired CO_2, heart rate, and electrocardiogram were monitored and maintained within physiologic limits. The spinal cord was severed by a laminectomy at T3 or T4. The nerve to the biceps femoris/semitendinosus muscles was dissected out and covered in mineral oil. One of the nerve filaments was placed on a recording electrode, and action potential discharge was counted using pulse integrators. A mechanical stimulus was applied to each foot every 5 minutes, and the total number of spikes elicited were counted. A baseline value for the reflex was calculated before any experimental manipulation. A chemical stimulus (mustard oil) was applied to a 4 mm^2 patch of skin on the dorsum of the foot. The sural and gastrocnemius nerves were electrically stimulated to produce central sensitization. The action potential discharge in flexor motor neurons was measured before and after administration of competitive and noncompetitive NMDA receptor antagonists.

Endpoints: The effect of NMDA receptor antagonists on central sensitization, as measured by changes in the excitability of the rat hind limb flexion withdrawal reflex.

RESULTS

- In the absence of experimental manipulation or treatment, a standard mechanical cutaneous stimulus produced a stable response (measured in terms of total number of action potentials generated in flexor motor neurons when repeated at 5-minute intervals over prolonged periods).

- Depending on dose, a reduction of the baseline reflex was observed with the administration of NMDA receptor antagonists.
- Stimulation of sural nerve C-fibers at 1 Hz produced an upward progression of action potentials elicited per stimulus over the 20-second period of stimulation (windup) as well as a period of reflex facilitation after the stimulation has ceased (maximal at 1 minute after the stimulus with return to baseline levels within 10 minutes).
- Systemic pretreatment with NMDA receptor antagonists prevented both windup and reflex facilitation from occurring during sural nerve stimulation.
- Using a chemical stimulus on the dorsum of the foot produces a prolonged period of increased excitability of the flexion reflex. Pretreatment with NMDA receptor antagonists prevented the induced reflex facilitation. After reflex facilitation was established, treatment with NMDA receptor antagonists returned the reflex to baseline levels.
- Stimulation of gastrocnemius nerve C-fibers produces a prolonged facilitation of the flexor reflex. The administration of an NMDA receptor antagonist 20 minutes after the induction of facilitation returned the reflex to baseline levels.

Criticisms and Limitations: This animal study raises the questions of what NMDA receptor antagonist doses would be required to inhibit facilitated pain signals and treat pain hypersensitivity in humans.

Other Relevant Studies and Information:

- A recent publication by Nielsen et al.[2] examined the use of intraoperative ketamine for spinal fusion surgery in chronic pain patients with opioid dependency. Compared with placebo, patients who received a ketamine bolus of 0.5 mg/kg followed by an infusion at 0.25 mg/kg/h during their procedures had significantly lower postoperative opioid consumption during the first 24 hours (patient-controlled analgesia [PCA] with intravenous morphine), decreased sedation in the first 6 to 24 hours postoperatively, and greater improvement in back pain at 6 months postoperatively compared with preoperative pain scores.
- A recent meta-analysis[3] of randomized trials examined whether ketamine added to morphine or hydromorphone PCA provides clinically relevant benefits. Analysis found that the addition of ketamine

to morphine or hydromorphone PCA provides a small improvement in postoperative analgesia while reducing opioid requirements and reduces postoperative nausea and vomiting without a detected increase in other adverse effects.

- In anesthesia practice, commonly used medications that are NMDA antagonists include ketamine, methadone, nitrous oxide, and tramadol.

Summary and Implications: This study demonstrated that the induction and maintenance of central sensitization are dependent on NMDA receptor activation. NMDA receptor antagonists have been shown to prevent the manifestation of central sensitization and to decrease established hyperactivity in pain pathways. NMDA receptor antagonists play an important role in pain management.

References

1. Woolf CJ, Thompson SW. The induction and maintenance of central sensitization is dependent on N-methyl-D-aspartic acid receptor activation: implications for the treatment of post-injury pain hypersensitivity states. *Pain.* 1991 Mar;44(3):293–99.
2. Nielsen RV, Fomsgaard JS, Siegel H, et al. Intraoperative ketamine reduces immediate postoperative opioid consumption after spinal fusion surgery in chronic pain patients with opioid dependency: a randomized, blinded trial. *Pain.* 2017 Mar;158(3):463–70.
3. Wang L, Johnston B, Kaushal A, Cheng D, Zhu F, Martin J. Ketamine added to morphine or hydromorphone patient-controlled analgesia for acute postoperative pain in adults: a systematic review and meta-analysis of randomized trials. *Can J Anaesth.* 2016 Mar;63(3):311–25.

37

Randomized Trial of Oral Morphine for Chronic Noncancer Pain

[Among patients with non-cancer-related chronic pain] and in whom there is no history of substance abuse . . . nine weeks of oral morphine . . . may be of analgesic benefit, but is unlikely to confer psychological or functional improvement . . . Further randomized controlled trials are required to define the role of oral morphine in the management of chronic non-cancer pain.

—MOULIN ET AL.[1]

Research Question: Do patients with chronic pain not due to cancer benefit from treatment with opioids?[1]

Funding: The Medical Research Council of Canada and Purdue Frederick, a pharmaceutical company that manufactures opioids.

Year Study Began: Mid-1990s.

Year Study Published: 1996.

Study Location: A pain clinic at Victoria Hospital in Ontario, Canada.

Who Was Studied: Adults 18–70 with stable non-cancer-related pain of ≥6 months' duration and of at least moderate intensity (≥5 on a 1–10 scale).

Patients were required to have "regional pain of a myofascial, musculoskeletal, or rheumatic nature." In addition, all study patients had failed to respond to nonsteroidal anti-inflammatory drugs and at least one month of tricyclic antidepressant therapy.

Who Was Excluded: Patients with a history of substance abuse, those with a history of psychosis or a major mood disorder, those with neuropathic pain syndromes such as reflex sympathetic dystrophy, those with isolated headache syndromes (since opioids may lead to rebound headaches), and those with other medical problems such as congestive heart failure that might complicate opioid therapy. In addition, patients were excluded if they had previously received opioids for chronic pain (prior codeine treatment was allowed, as codeine is available over-the-counter in Canada).

How Many Patients: 61.

Study Overview: See Figure 37.1 for an overview of the study's design.

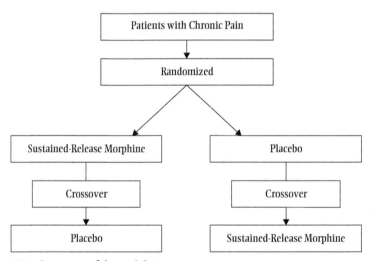

Figure 37.1 Summary of the trial design.

Study Intervention: Patients assigned to the morphine group received sustained-release morphine (MS Contin). The medication was titrated over 3 weeks, initially at a dose of 15 mg twice daily, up to a maximum of 60 mg twice daily if tolerated. The medication was then continued at the maximum tolerated dose for an additional 6 weeks before being tapered over 2 weeks.

Patients assigned to the placebo group received benztropine—a medication with "no analgesic properties" but that "mimics many of the possible side-effects of morphine." The benztropine was titrated in a similar fashion, initially at a dose of 0.25 mg twice daily up to a maximum of 1 mg twice daily if tolerated. Benztropine was then continued at the maximum tolerated dose for an additional 6 weeks before being tapered over 2 weeks.

At the completion of the taper, patients in both groups crossed over and received 11 weeks of the other therapy (i.e., all patients ultimately received 11 weeks of morphine and 11 weeks of placebo).

Patients in both groups could take paracetamol (acetaminophen) as a "rescue medication" when necessary. In addition, all study patients were offered group sessions led by a psychologist to learn "cognitive-behavioral strategies for pain management" (patients were not required to participate in these sessions).

Follow-Up: 11 weeks.

Endpoints: Primary outcome: patient-reported pain intensity on a 1–10 scale (1 = lowest intensity, 10 = highest intensity). Secondary outcomes: use of paracetamol for breakthrough pain; and scores on a panel of questionnaires measuring psychological and functional improvement.

RESULTS

- The mean age of study patients was 40 years, and the mean duration of pain symptoms was 4.1 years.
- 25% of the patients were employed, 85% had injury-related pain, and 41% had previously consulted five or more specialists about their pain.
- 38% of patients primarily suffered from head, neck, and shoulder pain, while 34% primarily suffered from back pain.
- The mean total daily dose of morphine tolerated by study patients was 83.5 mg.
- Patients in the morphine group had less pain than those in the placebo group, but psychological and functional outcomes were not significantly different between the groups (Tables 37.1 and 37.2).
- There appeared to be a "carryover effect," in which patients who received morphine during the first phase of the study had lower pain intensity scores during the second phase after being switched to placebo (the authors hypothesize that this may have been due to a persisting "psychological effect" from morphine).
- Patients in the morphine group were more likely than patients in the placebo group to experience vomiting (43% vs. 6%, $P = 0.0002$),

dizziness (50% vs. 15%, $P = 0.0004$), constipation (56% vs. 19%, $P = 0.0005$), and abdominal pain (29% vs. 11%, $P = 0.04$).

- 8.7% of patients in the morphine group vs. 4.3% in the placebo group reported drug craving (difference not significant).
- 41.3% of patients preferred treatment with morphine, 28.3% preferred treatment with placebo, and 30.4% had no preference ($P = 0.26$).

Table 37.1. PAIN INTENSITY SCORES (SCALE 1–10)*

Group	Baseline	9 Weeks[†]	11 Weeks[‡]	P Value[§]
Morphine	7.8	7.1	7.3	0.01
Placebo	7.8	7.9	8.5	

*These data are only from the first phase of the study before the crossover. Similar findings were noted when data from the second phase (after the crossover) were included.
[†]At the completion of full-dose treatment.
[‡]At the completion of the washout period.
[§]Comparison is for change in pain scores during phase 1 of the study in the morphine vs. placebo groups.

Table 37.2. OTHER OUTCOMES

Outcome	Morphine Group	Placebo Group	P Value
Tabs of paracetamol required per day for breakthrough pain	3.5	3.9	0.40
Psychological well-being*	67.7	67.7	Not significant[†]
Quality of life	24.5	24.2	Not significant[†]
Sickness Impact Profile[‡]	44.6	45.0	Not significant[†]
Pain Disability Index[§]			

*As assessed by the Symptom Check List-90, which is scored based on patient responses to a questionnaire from 30 to 81 "with higher scores indicating greater impairment."
[†]Actual P values not reported.
[‡]Scored based on patient responses to a questionnaire on a scale of 0–100 with "higher values indicating worse function."
[§]Scored based on patient responses to a questionnaire on a scale of 0–70 with "higher values indicating worse function."

Criticisms and Limitations: The patients were only followed for 11 weeks, and thus this study did not assess the long-term impact of opioid therapy.

Patients in this study were monitored very closely (they had visits with the study team every 1–2 weeks). It is uncertain whether opioid therapy would have the same effects in a less closely monitored setting more typical of a "real-world" environment.

Patients with substance abuse disorders were excluded from the study, and thus the results do not apply to these patients.

Other Relevant Studies and Information:

- There have been surprisingly few other studies evaluating the use of opioids for the treatment of chronic noncancer pain. Most other studies were also small, had a follow-up of <16 weeks, and compared opioids with placebo (rather than with another active therapy). These studies have generally come to similar conclusions as this study, namely that opioids lead to a modest reduction in pain scores and, at best, a small improvement in functional outcomes.[2,3]
- Opioids are widely felt to be appropriate for chronic use in patients with pain due to cancer and other life-threatening conditions, and many experts believe that opioids are underprescribed among these patients.
- Opioids have become one of the most widely used medications in the United States.[4]
- Guidelines from the American Pain Society state that "although evidence is limited . . . chronic opioid therapy can be an effective therapy for carefully selected and monitored patients with chronic non-cancer pain. However, opioids are also associated with potentially serious harms, including opioid-related adverse effects and outcomes related to the abuse potential of opioids."[5]

Summary and Implications: Among patients with non–cancer-related pain, sustained-release oral morphine led to a modest reduction in pain but no clear improvement in psychological or functional outcomes. Patients in the morphine group experienced an increased rate of gastrointestinal symptoms and dizziness. The study had important methodologic limitations, most notably that patients were only followed for 11 weeks. In addition, patients with a history of substance abuse were excluded, limiting the generalizability of the findings. Despite these limitations, this study represents one of the highest quality studies to evaluate opioids for chronic noncancer pain.

CLINICAL CASE: OPIOIDS FOR NONCANCER PAIN

Case History

A 28-year-old woman presents to your clinic after returning from combat in Afghanistan with chronic neck pain. Her symptoms began after a whiplash injury suffered during combat. The pain has persisted for almost a year and substantially interferes with her life. She reports difficulty sleeping due to the pain and says that the pain reaches at least 7 on a scale from 1–10 most days of the week. She has tried over-the-counter pain medications, including acetaminophen and ibuprofen, but these medications "barely take the edge off."

The patient tells you that her friend was recently given morphine and Vicodin (acetaminophen and hydrocodone) for back pain, and this seems to have helped. The patient wonders whether she might benefit from these medications as well. What can you tell her based on the results of this study?

Suggested Answer

This patient has chronic, non–cancer-related pain that substantially interferes with her life. Studies evaluating opioids for chronic non–cancer-related pain indicate that these medications may reduce pain in the short term. However, data on outcomes after 16 weeks are scant, and the impact of opioids on psychological and functional outcomes are uncertain. In addition, opioids lead to significant side effects and potentially to addiction in some high-risk patients. For these reasons, nonopioid treatment options should be fully explored before starting chronic opioid therapy.

The patient in this vignette has tried over-the-counter pain medications but should also try nonpharmacologic strategies for pain management such as physical therapy or cognitive-behavioral therapy. If these strategies prove ineffective, you might consider a long-acting medication for chronic pain such as amitriptyline. In the meantime, the patient could continue using nonnarcotic pain relievers such as acetaminophen and ibuprofen. It would also be reasonable to prescribe a small supply of a short-acting opioid medication such as an acetaminophen and hydrocodone combination (Vicodin) for episodes of severe pain. (The patient might use this medication when she has difficulty sleeping.)

If nonopioid therapy is ultimately ineffective, it would be appropriate to consider opioid therapy (others might reasonably decide not to use opioids in a patient such as this, however). If the decision to initiate opioids is made, it would first be necessary to evaluate risk factors for substance abuse. In addition, the patient should agree to a pain contract stating that opioids are only to be prescribed by one provider (usually the primary care provider or a pain specialist) as well as other stipulations to ensure safe use.

References

1. Moulin DE, Iezzi A, Amireh R, et al. Randomised trial of oral morphine for chronic non-cancer pain. *Lancet.* 1996;347:143–47.
2. Kalso E, Edwards JE, Moore RA, McQuay HJ. Opioids in chronic non-cancer pain: systematic review of efficacy and safety. *Pain.* 2004;112(3):372–80.
3. Furlan AD, Sandoval JA, Mailis-Gagnon A, Tunks E. Opioids for chronic noncancer pain: a meta-analysis of effectiveness and side effects. *CMAJ.* 2006;174(11):1589–94.
4. Okie S. A flood of opioids, a rising tide of deaths. *N Engl J Med.* 2011;364(4):290.
5. American Pain Society. *Guideline for the use of opioid therapy in chronic noncancer pain: evidence review.* Glenview, IL: American Pain Society, 2009.

38

Epidural Glucocorticoid Injections for Spinal Stenosis

In the treatment of lumbar spinal stenosis, epidural injection of glucocorticoids plus lidocaine offered minimal or no short-term benefit as compared with epidural injection of lidocaine alone.

—FRIEDLY ET AL.[1]

Research Question: What is the effectiveness of epidural injections of glucocorticoids plus anesthetic compared with injections of anesthetic alone in patients with lumbar spinal stenosis?

Funding: Agency for Healthcare Research and Quality.

Year Study Began: 2011.

Year Study Published: 2014.

Study Location: 16 sites in the United States.

Who Was Studied: Adult patients ≥50 years of age with evidence of central lumbar spinal stenosis on magnetic resonance imaging or computed tomography and an average pain rating >4 (on a 0-to-10 scale with 0 = no pain and 10 = worst possible pain) in the lower back, buttock, leg, or a combination of these sites on standing, walking, or spinal extension in the week before enrollment. Pain in the buttock, leg, or both had to be greater than in the back, and a score ≥7 on the Roland-Morris Disability Questionnaire (RMDQ) (range of 0–24, with higher scores indicative of greater disability) was required.

Who Was Excluded: Patients with a history of lumbar surgery, epidural glucocorticoid injections within the previous 6 months, or spondylolisthesis requiring surgery.

How Many Patients: 400.

Study Overview: See Figure 38.1 for an overview of the study's design.

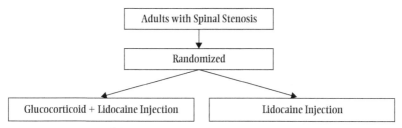

Figure 38.1 Summary of the study design.

Study Intervention: In this double-blind trial, patients received one or two standardized epidural injections with fluoroscopic guidance during a 6-week period. The approach for injections (interlaminar or transforaminal) was chosen at the physician's discretion. Patients were randomized to receive an epidural injection of glucocorticoid plus lidocaine (200 patients) vs. lidocaine alone (200 patients). Patients in the glucocorticoid group received 1 to 3 mL of triamcinolone (60–120 mg), betamethasone (6–12 mg), dexamethasone (8–10 mg), or methylprednisolone (60–120 mg). The lidocaine component consisted of 1 to 3 mL of 0.25% to 1% lidocaine. Adverse events were documented during or immediately after the procedure. All outcomes and morning serum cortisol levels were assessed at baseline, 3 weeks, and 6 weeks after randomization. Patients were able to receive a repeat injection at 3 weeks if they wished.

Follow-Up: 6 weeks.

Endpoints: Primary outcomes measured at 6 weeks: the RMDQ score and the patient's rating of buttock, hip, or leg pain averaged over the previous week. Secondary outcomes: proportion of patients with at least minimal (≥30%) and substantial (≥50%) clinically meaningful improvement from baseline to

6 weeks; ratings of average back pain in the previous week; scores on the Brief Pain Inventory (BPI); scores on the eight-question version of the Patient Health Questionnaire (PHQ-8); scores on the Generalized Anxiety Disorder 7 (GAD-7) scale; scores on the European Quality of Life-5 Dimensions (EQ-5D) questionnaire; scores on the Swiss Spinal Stenosis Questionnaire (SSSQ); physical function scores; satisfaction with treatment scores.

RESULTS

- Baseline patient characteristics were similar between the two study groups except for an imbalance with respect to duration of pain.
- At 3 weeks, the glucocorticoid group showed greater improvement than the lidocaine group in RMDQ scores and intensity of leg pain, but the differences were clinically insignificant based on the percent improvement in RMDQ from baseline.
- At 6 weeks, both groups demonstrated improvement in the RMDQ score compared with baseline, but there was no significant difference in the average treatment effect, intensity of leg pain, BPI, SSSQ symptoms and physical function, EQ-5D, or GAD-7 scales between the two groups. After adjustment for duration of pain, the glucocorticoid group had significantly greater improvement in the RMDQ score, but the difference was small.
- The glucocorticoid group had greater improvement in symptoms of depression on the PHQ-8 scale $(P = 0.007)$ and was more satisfied with treatment $(P = 0.01)$.
- For transforaminal injections, there were no significant differences between groups in any outcome at 3 or 6 weeks. For interlaminar injections, there was significantly better physical function on the RMDQ and less leg pain at 3 weeks in the glucocorticoid vs. the lidocaine group; there was no difference between the two groups at 6 weeks.
- The difference in proportion of patients experiencing adverse events between groups was not significant, but there were more adverse events on average per person in the glucocorticoid group compared with the lidocaine group $(P = 0.02)$, with a higher rate among patients who received transforaminal injections.
- At both 3 and 6 weeks, a significantly higher proportion of patients in the glucocorticoid plus lidocaine group had morning serum cortisol levels less than 3 mcg/dL or less than 10 mcg/dL compared with the lidocaine group.

Criticisms and Limitations: Patients with prior lumbar surgery were excluded, limiting the generalizability of the findings. The study did not randomly assign patients to the injection approach (transforaminal vs. interlaminar).

Other Relevant Studies and Information:

- A meta-analysis of 13 randomized controlled trials comparing the effectiveness of epidural injections of anesthetic with and without steroids for the treatment of spinal stenosis found the inclusion of steroids to confer no advantage to local anesthetic alone; epidural injections with steroids or with local anesthetic alone provide significant pain relief and functional improvement.[2]
- The American Society of Anesthesiologists (ASA) Practice Guidelines for Chronic Pain Management[3] state that "epidural steroid injections with or without local anesthetics may be used as part of a multimodal treatment regimen to provide pain relief in selected patients with radicular pain or radiculopathy."
- A systematic review and meta-analysis published in 2013 evaluated whether epidural nonsteroid injections for spinal pain constitute a treatment or true placebo in comparison with nonepidural injections for the treatment of back and neck pain. Only a few trials directly compared epidural nonsteroid with nonepidural injections, and these trials showed no benefit. Indirect comparisons of the techniques from a larger number of trials suggested that epidural nonsteroid injections conferred some benefit and were more likely than nonepidural injections to achieve positive outcomes and provide greater pain reduction.[4]

Summary and Implications: This study demonstrated that epidural injection containing glucocorticoids for the treatment of lumbar stenosis offered minimal or no benefit over epidural injection of lidocaine alone at 6 weeks. Systemic absorption of glucocorticoids and suppression of the hypothalamic-pituitary axis was demonstrated among patients who received epidural injections containing glucocorticoids.

References

1. Friedly JL, Comstock BA, Turner JA, et al. A randomized trial of epidural glucocorticoid injections for spinal stenosis. *N Engl J Med.* 2014 Jul 3;371(1):11–21.
2. Meng H, Fei Q, Wang B, et al. Epidural injections with or without steroids in managing chronic low back pain secondary to lumbar spinal stenosis: a meta-analysis of 13 randomized controlled trials. *Drug Des Devel Ther.* 2015 Aug 13;9:4657–67.

3. American Society of Anesthesiologists Task Force on Chronic Pain Management, American Society of Regional Anesthesia and Pain Medicine. Practice guidelines for chronic pain management: an updated report by the American Society of Anesthesiologists Task Force on Chronic Pain Management and the American Society of Regional Anesthesia and Pain Medicine. *Anesthesiology.* 2010 Apr;112(4):810–33.

4. Bicket MC, Gupta A, Brown CH 4th, Cohen SP. Epidural injections for spinal pain: a systematic review and meta-analysis evaluating the "control" injections in randomized controlled trials. *Anesthesiology.* 2013 Oct;119(4):907–31.

39

Magnetic Resonance Imaging of the Lumbar Spine in People Without Back Pain

Although . . . patients preferred [rapid MRI scans to plain radiographs for the evaluation of low back pain], substituting rapid MRI for radiographic evaluations . . . may offer little additional benefit to patients, and it may increase the costs of care because of the increased number of spine operations that patients are likely to undergo.

—Jarvik et al.[1]

Research Question: Should patients with low back pain requiring imaging be offered plain radiographs or magnetic resonance imaging (MRI)?[1]

Funding: The Agency for Healthcare Research and Quality and the National Institute for Arthritis and Musculoskeletal and Skin Diseases.

Year Study Began: 1998.

Year Study Published: 2003.

Study Location: Four imaging sites in Washington State (an outpatient clinic, a teaching hospital, a multispecialty clinic, and a private imaging center).

Who Was Studied: Adults 18 years and older referred by their physician for radiographs of the lumbar spine to evaluate lower back pain and/or radiculopathy.

Who Was Excluded: Patients with lumbar surgery within the previous year, those with acute external trauma, and those with metallic implants in the spine.

How Many Patients: 380.

Study Overview: See Figure 39.1 for an overview of the study's design.

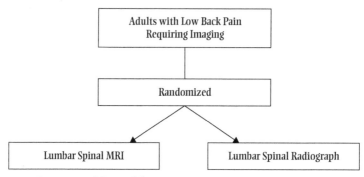

Figure 39.1 Summary of the trial design.

Study Intervention: Patients assigned to the plain radiograph group received the films according to standard protocol. Most patients received anteroposterior and lateral views only; however, a small number received additional views when requested by the ordering physician.

Patients assigned to the MRI group were scheduled for the scan on the day of study enrollment whenever possible, and if not, within a week of enrollment. Most scans were performed with a field strength of 1.5 T, and all patients received sagittal and axial T2-weighted images.

Follow-Up: 12 months.

Endpoints: Primary outcome: scores on the 23-item modified Roland-Morris back pain disability scale.[2] Secondary outcomes: quality of life as assessed using the Medical Outcomes Study 36-Item Short Form Survey (SF-36)[3]; patient satisfaction with care as assessed using the Deyo-Diehl patient satisfaction questionnaire[4]; days of lost work; patient reassurance; and health care resource utilization.

The 23-item modified Roland-Morris back pain disability scale consists of 23 "yes" or "no" questions. Patients are given one point for each "yes" answer for a total possible score of 23. Below are sample questions on the scale:

- I stay at home most of the time because of my back problem or leg pain (sciatica).

- I walk more slowly than usual because of my back problem or leg pain (sciatica).
- I stay in bed most of the time because of my back or leg pain (sciatica).

RESULTS

- The mean age of study patients was 53; 15% were either unemployed, disabled, or on leave from work; 24% had depression; and 70% reported pain radiating to the legs.
- 49% of patients were referred for imaging by primary care doctors, while 51% were referred by specialists.
- The spinal MRI revealed disk herniation in 33% of patients, nerve root impingement in 7%, moderate or severe central canal stenosis in 20%, and lateral recess stenosis in 17%—findings that are typically not detectable with plain radiographs.
- There were no significant differences in back pain scores between the radiograph and MRI groups, although patients in the MRI group were more likely to be reassured by their imaging results; there were no significant differences in total health care costs between the groups (Tables 39.1 and 39.2).

Table 39.1. THE TRIAL'S KEY FINDINGS AFTER 12 MONTHS*

Outcome	Radiograph Group	MRI Group	P Value
Roland-Morris Back Pain Score (scale: 0–23)[†]	8.75	9.34	0.53
SF-36, physical functioning (scale: 0–100)[‡]	63.77	61.04	Not significant[§]
Patient satisfaction (scale: 0–11)[‡]	7.34	7.04	Not significant[§]
Days of lost work in past 4 weeks	1.26	1.57	Not significant[§]
Were you reassured by the imaging results?	58%	74%	0.002

*The 12-month outcomes were adjusted for baseline scores, for example, the 12-month Roland scores were adjusted for the fact that, at baseline, scores were slightly higher in patients randomized to the MRI group.
[†]Higher scores indicate a worse outcome.
[‡]Higher scores indicate a better outcome.
[§]Actual P value not reported.

Table 39.2. COMPARISON OF RESOURCE UTILIZATION DURING THE STUDY PERIOD

Outcome	Radiograph Group	MRI Group	P Value
Patients receiving opioid analgesics	25%	26%	0.94
Subsequent MRIs per patient	0.22	0.09	0.01
Physical therapy, acupuncture, and massage visits per patient	7.9	3.8	0.008
Specialist consultations per patient	0.49	0.73	0.07
Patients receiving lumbar spine surgery	2%	6%	0.09
Total costs of health care services	$1,651	$2,121	0.11

Criticisms and Limitations: The increased rate of spinal surgeries and the higher cost of health care services in the MRI group did not reach statistical significance. Therefore, it is not appropriate to draw firm conclusions from these findings.

Other Relevant Studies and Information:

- Other trials have suggested that early spinal imaging (radiographs, computed tomography, and MRI) does not improve outcomes in patients with acute lower back pain without alarm symptoms such as worsening neurologic function,[5] nor does it substantially assist with decision making in patients referred for epidural steroid injections of the spine.[6]
- Guidelines[7] recommend that MRI of the lumbar spine only be obtained in patients with signs or symptoms of:
  - Emergent conditions such as the cauda equina syndrome, tumors, infections, or fractures with neurologic impingement.
  - Radicular symptoms severe enough and long-lasting enough to warrant surgical intervention.
  - Spinal stenosis severe enough and long-lasting enough to warrant surgical intervention.

Summary and Implications: Although spinal MRI studies (compared with plain radiographs) are reassuring for patients with low back pain, they do not lead to improved functional outcomes. In addition, spinal MRI detects anatomic abnormalities that would otherwise go undiscovered, possibly leading to spinal surgeries of uncertain value.

CLINICAL CASE: MRI FOR LOW BACK PAIN

Case History

A 52-year-old man with 6 weeks of low back pain visits your office requesting an MRI of his spine. His symptoms began after doing yard work and have improved only slightly during this time period. The pain is bothersome, but not incapacitating, and radiates down his right leg. He has no systemic symptoms (fevers, chills, or weight loss) and denies bowel or bladder dysfunction. He reports difficulty walking because of the pain. On examination, he is an over-weight man in no apparent distress. His range of motion is limited because of pain. He has no neurologic deficits.

Based on the results of this trial, should you order an MRI for this patient?

Suggested Answer

Based on the results of this trial, ordering a spinal MRI in a patient like the one in this vignette is unlikely to lead to improved functional outcomes and may increase the likelihood of spinal surgery by detecting anatomic abnor-malities that would otherwise go undiscovered. Still, this trial showed that an MRI may provide reassurance to patients. For this reason, you should re-assure your patient in other ways, for example, by telling him that he does not have any signs or symptoms of a serious back problem like an infection or cancer.

Other types of spinal imaging such as plain radiographs do not appear to im-prove outcomes in patients with acute low back pain without alarm symptoms either. Thus, even a plain film may not be necessary at this time.

References

1. Jarvik JG, Hollingworth W, Martin B, et al. Rapid magnetic resonance imaging vs radiographs for patients with low back pain: a randomized controlled trial. *JAMA*. 2003;289(21):2810–8.
2. Roland M, Morris R. A study of the natural history of back pain, 1: development of a reliable and sensitive measure of disability in low back pain. *Spine*. 1983;8:141–44.
3. Ware JE, Sherbourne CD. The MOS 36-item short-form survey (SF-36), I: concep-tual framework and item selection. *Med Care*. 1992;30:473–83.
4. Deyo RA, Diehl AK. Patient satisfaction with medical care for low-back pain. *Spine*. 1986;11:28–30.
5. Chou R, Fu R, Carrino JA, Deyo RA. Imaging strategies for low-back pain: system-atic review and meta-analysis. *Lancet*. 2009;373(9662):463.

6. Cohen SP, Gupta A, Strassels SA, et al. Effect of MRI on treatment results or decision making in patients with lumbosacral radiculopathy referred for epidural steroid injections: a multicenter, randomized controlled trial. *Arch Intern Med.* 2012;172(2):134.

7. Bigos SJ, et al. *Acute low back pain problems in adults.* Clinical practice guideline No 14. Rockville, MD: Agency for Health Care Policy and Research, Public Health Service, US Department of Health and Human Services, December 1994.

40

Surgery vs. Rehabilitation for Chronic Lower Back Pain

Patients with low back pain . . . may obtain similar benefits from an intensive rehabilitation programme as they do from surgery.

—FAIRBANK ET AL.[1]

Research Question: Is spinal fusion surgery beneficial in patients with chronic nonspecific low back pain?[1]

Funding: The Medical Research Council of the United Kingdom.

Year Study Began: 1996.

Year Study Published: 2005.

Study Location: 15 centers in the United Kingdom.

Who Was Studied: Adults 18–55 years old with at least 12 months of chronic low back pain (with or without referred pain).

Who Was Excluded: Patients who were poor candidates for either of the two treatment strategies; for example, patients with spinal infections who required surgery. In addition, patients with previous spinal surgery were excluded.

How Many Patients: 349.

Study Overview: See Figure 40.1 for an overview of the study's design.

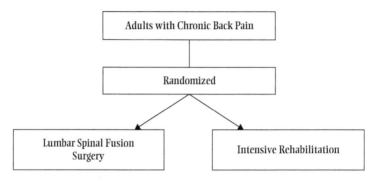

Figure 40.1 Summary of the MRC Spine Stabilization Trial design.

Study Intervention: Patients assigned to the surgery group underwent spinal fusion surgery. The surgical technique (e.g., the approach, implant, cages, and bone graft material) "was left to the discretion of the surgeon."

Patients assigned to the intensive rehabilitation group were assigned to a 3-week outpatient education and exercise program. The program varied by site but typically involved 75 hours of therapy along with a follow-up session several weeks afterward. Physiotherapists led the sessions, and psychologists assisted at most sites as well. In addition, the instructors "used principles of cognitive behavior therapy to identify and overcome fears and unhelpful beliefs that many patients develop when in pain." Patients who did not have an adequate response to rehabilitation were offered surgery.

Follow-Up: 24 months.

Endpoints: Primary outcomes: Patient-reported pain on the Oswestry low back pain disability index; and patient performance on the shuttle walk test. Secondary outcomes: scores on the short form 36 (SF-36) general health questionnaire; and surgical complications.

- The Oswestry low back pain disability index is scored from 0 (no disability) to 100 (completely disabled or bedridden).[2] In the shuttle walk test, the distance patients walk during a specified time period and while following instructions is recorded.[3]

RESULTS

- Among patients assigned to the surgery group, 79% received surgery during the study period (21% of patients presumably declined surgery).
- Among patients assigned to the rehabilitation group, 28% received surgery during the study period either because of patient request or because of an inadequate response to rehabilitation.
- 12% of patients who underwent surgery experienced a complication such as excessive bleeding, a dural tear, or a vascular injury.
- 8% of patients who received surgery required additional surgery after the first operation either to treat a surgical complication or because of persistent symptoms.
- Although scores on the Oswestry back pain scale were significantly better in the surgery group compared with the rehabilitation group, the difference was very small and is of questionable clinical importance (Table 40.1).

Table 40.1. SUMMARY OF THE TRIAL'S KEY FINDINGS

Outcome	Change in Score During Study Period, Surgery Group	Change in Score During Study Period, Rehabilitation Group	P Value*
Oswestry Back Pain Score[+]	−12.5	−8.7	0.045
Shuttle Walking Test[+]	+98 meters	+63 meters	0.12
SF-36[§]			
Physical Score	+9.4	+7.6	0.21
Mental Score	+4.2	+3.9	0.90

*P value is adjusted for baseline differences between the groups.
[+]A reduction in the back pain score indicates an improvement.
[+]An increase in walking distance on the shuttle walk test indicates an improvement.
[§]An increase in the SF-36 score indicates an improvement.

Criticisms and Limitations: Approximately 20% of patients in the study were lost to follow-up. In addition, there was considerable crossover between the groups (21% of patients in the surgical group never received the surgery, while 28% of patients in the rehabilitation group did receive surgery).

The rehabilitation program used in this study was very intensive and might be too expensive or impractical for many patients. However, whether this intensive rehabilitation program is superior to less intensive programs—or to no rehabilitation at all—is not known.

In the surgery group, the surgical technique was left to the discretion of the surgeon. Surgical outcomes might have been better if the surgical technique had been standardized, though there is considerable controversy about which surgical techniques are best.

Other Relevant Studies and Information:

- Three other trials have compared surgery with nonsurgical treatment for chronic low back pain; however, none was of high methodologic quality. A meta-analysis of data from these three trials and the MRC Trial concluded: "Surgery may be more efficacious than unstructured nonsurgical care for chronic back pain but may not be more efficacious than structured cognitive-behavior therapy. Methodological limitations of the randomized trials prevent firm conclusions."[4]
- Recently, a new surgical technique has been developed for treating patients with chronic low back pain: lumbar disk replacement with an artificial disk. Studies have demonstrated slight improvements with disk replacement compared with nonoperative care, but the clinical importance of this small difference is uncertain, and it is unclear whether the risks of surgery outweigh the small benefit.[5,6]
- A number of trials have compared surgery (diskectomy) with nonsurgical treatment in patients with severe, persistent sciatica. These trials have generally shown equivalent surgical and nonsurgical outcomes after a year but slightly faster improvement in the surgical group.[7]
- Guidelines from the American Pain Society recommend that patients with disabling lower back pain lasting more than a year be informed of the risks and benefits of both surgical and nonsurgical treatment options. Because both treatments may be equally effective in the long term, the decision about which treatment to pursue should be made by the patient.[8]

Summary and Implications: The benefit of surgery compared with nonsurgical therapy in patients with chronic low back pain remains uncertain. Most patients improve both with and without surgery. Although pain control may be slightly better with surgery, surgical treatment carries risks. Further research on this topic is greatly needed.

CLINICAL CASE: CHRONIC LOW BACK PAIN

Case History

A 48-year-old man with low back pain for the past several years is referred to an orthopedic surgeon to consider surgical treatment with lumbar spinal fusion. The symptoms began gradually and can be quite bothersome; however, they do not interfere with his ability to work. The patient denies weakness or bowel or bladder dysfunction. The pain is partially relieved with nonsteroidal anti-inflammatory medications.

On physical examination, the patient is obese (body mass index of 33). He has a normal neurological examination, and on the straight leg raise test, his back pain does not radiate below his knees.

He requests your advice about whether or not to pursue surgery. He feels anxious about "going under the knife" but is willing to do it if you think it will help him. Based on the results of the MRC Spine Stabilization Trial, how should you advise him?

Suggested Answer

The benefits of surgical therapy for chronic low back pain remain uncertain. While existing trials suggest that surgery may lead to slightly improved pain control compared with nonsurgical therapy, the benefits appear to be small. In addition, surgical treatment carries risks. For these reasons, patients with chronic debilitating low back pain should be informed of the risks and benefits of both surgical and nonsurgical treatment options. Using this information, patients should choose the treatment that is most compatible with their personal preferences.

The patient in this vignette has chronic low back pain, but his symptoms do not appear to be debilitating. In addition, his symptoms may improve with weight loss. Moreover, he reports feeling anxious about surgery. For these reasons, he is currently not a good surgical candidate.

If this patient's symptoms worsen, however, surgical treatment could be considered. Before undergoing surgery, he should be informed of the risks and benefits. In addition, he should be informed that his pain will likely improve considerably over time, even without surgery. The ultimate decision about whether or not to proceed should rest with the patient.

References

1. Fairbank J, Frost H, Wilson-MacDonald J, et al. Randomised controlled trial to compare surgical stabilization of the lumbar spine with an intensive rehabilitation programme for patients with chronic lower back pain: the MRC spine stabilisation trial. *BMJ*. 2005;330(7502):1233.
2. Fairbank JC, Pynsent PB. The Oswestry disability index. *Spine (Phila Pa 1976)*. 2000;25:2940–53.
3. Taylor S, Frost H, Taylor A, Barker K. Reliability and responsiveness of the shuttle walking test in patients with chronic lower back pain. *Physiother Res Int*. 2001;6:170–78.
4. Mirza SK, Deyo RA. Systematic review of randomized trials comparing lumbar fusion surgery to nonoperative care for treatment of chronic back pain. *Spine (Phila Pa 1976)*. 2007;32(7):816–23.
5. Hellum C, Johnsen LG, Storheim K, et al. Surgery with disc prosthesis vs. rehabilitation in patients with low back pain and degenerative disc: two year follow-up of randomised study. *BMJ*. 2011;342:d2786.
6. Jacobs WC, van der Gaag NA, Kruyt MC, et al. Total disc replacement for chronic discogenic low back pain: a Cochrane review. *Spine (Phila Pa 1976)*. 2013;38(1):24.
7. Peul WC, van Houwelingen HC, van den Hout WB, et al. Surgery versus prolonged conservative treatment for sciatica. *N Engl J Med*. 2007;356(22):2245–56.
8. Chou R, Loeser JD, Owens DK, et al. Interventional therapies, surgery, and interdisciplinary rehabilitation for low back pain: an evidence-based clinical practice guideline from the American Pain Society. *Spine (Phila Pa 1976)*. 2009;34(10):1066–77.

41

Preoperative Multimodal Analgesia for Laparoscopic Cholecystectomy

The concomitant use of local anesthetic and nonsteroidal anti-inflammatory and opioid drugs proved to be highly effective in our patients, resulting in faster recovery and discharge.
—MICHALOLIAKOU ET AL.[1]

Research Question: Does prophylactic multimodal nociceptive blockade delay the onset of postoperative pain, decrease analgesic requirements, speed recovery, and facilitate same-day discharge in patients undergoing elective laparoscopic cholecystectomy?

Funding: Ministry of Health in Greece.

Year Study Published: 1996.

Study Location: Toronto Hospital, University of Toronto, Toronto, Ontario, Canada.

Who Was Studied: American Society of Anesthesiologists (ASA) physical status I and II patients between 18 and 60 years of age undergoing elective laparoscopic cholecystectomy.

Who Was Excluded: Patients with significant cardiac, respiratory, hepatic, renal, or hematologic disorders; contraindications to administration of the study drugs; histories including gastrointestinal bleeding, monoamine oxidase inhibitor therapy, or alcohol abuse; prior upper abdominal or recent surgery; preexisting pain.

How Many Patients: 49.

Study Overview: See Figure 41.1 for an overview of the study's design.

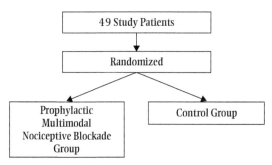

Figure 41.1 Summary of the study design.

Study Intervention: Intraoperative anesthetic care and postoperative pain and nausea management were standardized for all patients. Forty-five minutes before induction, the treatment group was premedicated with intramuscular (IM) meperidine and ketorolac, while the control group received two IM injections of placebo (normal saline). Ten minutes before incision, local anesthetic (treatment group) or normal saline (control group) was infiltrated into the skin at the site of skin incision, the subcutaneous tissue overlying the peritoneum at the site of skin puncture, and around the gallbladder. Both groups received intravenous (IV) metoclopramide 20 minutes before the end of surgery. Pain and nausea were assessed preoperatively, on arrival to and discharge from the postanesthesia care unit (PACU), and at 30 minutes and 1, 2, 3, 4, 10, 24, and 48 hours postoperatively.

Follow-Up: 48 hours postoperatively.

Endpoints: Time until patient was oriented to person, place, and time; time from PACU admission to first request for analgesic medication; time to reach PACU discharge criteria; total amount of meperidine, ketorolac, and dimenhydrinate administered and number of patients requiring these medications; time to tolerate oral fluids and solid food; time to void; time to ambulation; time to hospital discharge.

RESULTS

- Four patients, three from the treatment group and one from the control group, were excluded from the study analysis because of surgical complications. Study groups were similar in terms of patient age, gender, weight, ASA class, baseline and preinduction pain and nausea scores, duration of surgery, and total dose of propofol received.
- Intraoperatively, the treatment group received significantly less fentanyl than the control group ($P < 0.05$).
- On PACU arrival, the treatment group had significantly more patients without pain (57% vs. 4%), and the severity of pain was sixfold less compared with the control group. Pain scores were significantly lower at all measurement intervals in the treatment group than in the control group until 24 hours postoperatively.
- Postoperatively, significantly fewer patients required meperidine or ketorolac in the treatment group, resulting in lower total mean analgesic consumption. The time to first analgesic request was 6 hours in the treatment group vs. 20 minutes in the control group.
- Four patients in the control group developed Spo_2 <92% after receiving IV meperidine for pain in the PACU and required increased use of supplemental O_2.
- The duration of PACU stay and times to first sit-up, oral intake, and ambulation were significantly shorter in the treatment group compared with the control group.
- Of the treatment patients, 90.5% were discharged as ambulatory patients compared with 70.8% of control patients. Functional activity at 48 hours was significantly higher in the treatment group compared with the control group ($P < 0.05$).

Criticisms and Limitations: This study applies only to the narrow group of patients included (ASA physical status I and II patients between 18 and 60 years of age undergoing elective laparoscopic cholecystectomy). This study was conducted before the US Food and Drug Administration issuing a black box warning for droperidol in 2001.

Other Relevant Studies and Information:

- Using regional or neuraxial techniques as part of multimodal analgesia reduces the neurohumoral response to surgical stress.[2]
- Enhanced Recovery After Surgery (ERAS) protocols are multimodal perioperative care pathways designed to improve outcomes after surgical procedures, with key elements being preoperative counseling, nutritional optimization, multimodal analgesia, and early mobilization. There is a significant body of evidence that ERAS protocols lead to improved outcomes while shortening the duration of hospitalization and reducing costs.[3]
- The ASA Practice Guidelines for Acute Pain Management in the Perioperative Setting recommend multimodal techniques for pain management whenever possible. "Unless contraindicated, patients should receive an around-the-clock regimen of NSAIDs [nonsteroidal anti-inflammatory drugs], COXIBs [cyclooxygenase-2 inhibitors], or acetaminophen. Regional blockade with local anesthetics should be considered."[4]

Summary and Implications: This randomized, double-blind study demonstrated the benefit of preoperative multimodal analgesia on recovery and discharge.

CLINICAL CASE: MULTIMODAL ANALGESIA

Case History
A 52-year-old woman with colon cancer presents on day of surgery for laparotomy and total colectomy. The patient is obese (body mass index of 37) and has obstructive sleep apnea. Given the patient's past medical history and planned surgical procedure, how should this patient's pain be managed in order to optimize perioperative analgesia and promote recovery?

Suggested Answer
Multimodal analgesia should be pursued, and long-acting benzodiazepines and opiates should be minimized. The patient should be offered regional or neuraxial blockade preoperatively. Intraoperatively, unless contraindicated, a multimodal analgesic strategy may include the use of ketamine, acetaminophen,

NSAIDs, and short-acting IV narcotics (if needed). Postoperatively, regional or neuraxial analgesia should be optimized and supplemented with an opioid-sparing multimodal regimen.

References

1. Michaloliakou C, Chung F, Sharma S. Preoperative multimodal analgesia facilitates recovery after ambulatory laparoscopic cholecystectomy. *Anesth Analg.* 1996 Jan;82(1):44–51.
2. Kehlet H, Holte K. Effect of postoperative analgesia on surgical outcome. *Br J Anaesth.* 2001 Jul;87(1):62–72.
3. Stone AB, Grant MC, Pio Roda C, et al. Implementation costs of an Enhanced Recovery After Surgery Program in the United States: a financial model and sensitivity analysis based on a experiences at a quaternary academic medical center. *J Am Coll Surg.* 2016 Mar;222(3):219–25.
4. American Society of Anesthesiologists Task Force on Acute Pain Management. Practice guidelines for acute pain management in the perioperative setting: an updated report by the American Society of Anesthesiologists Task Force on Acute Pain Management. *Anesthesiology.* 2012 Feb;116(2):248–73.

Regional Anesthesiology

42

Neuraxial Anesthesia and Postoperative Mortality and Morbidity

Neuraxial blockade reduces postoperative mortality and other serious complications. The size of some of these benefits remains uncertain, and further research is required to determine whether these effects are due solely to benefits of neuraxial blockade or partly to avoidance of general anaesthesia. Nevertheless, these findings support more widespread use of neuraxial blockade.

—Rodgers et al.[1]

Research Question: What are the effects of neuraxial blockade with epidural or spinal anesthesia on postoperative morbidity and mortality?

Funding: Health Research Council of New Zealand and Astra Pain, New Zealand.

Year Study Published: Results of individual trials were published during the 1970s, 1980s, and 1990s. This review was published in 2000.

Study Location: University of Auckland, Auckland, New Zealand.

Who Was Studied: This systematic review examined all trials with random-ization to intraoperative neuraxial blockade (with epidural or spinal anes-thesia) or no neuraxial blockade for which data were available before January 1, 1997.

Who Was Excluded: Of the 158 potentially eligible trials, 10 trials were excluded because they were quasi-randomized (such as assignment according to date of birth), six trials were excluded because not all participants were randomized, and one trial was excluded because the groups differed with respect to heparin treat-ment and anesthetic technique.

How Many Patients: 9,559 patients over 141 included trials.

Study Overview: See Figure 42.1 for an overview of the study's design.

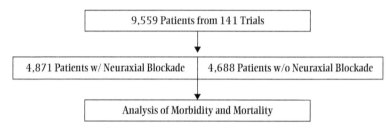

Figure 42.1 Summary of the study design.

Study Intervention: A computerized search using multiple electronic databases was conducted. A standard data collection sheet was used to record details of each trial (design, interventions, patient characteristics, and events). Two reviewers independently recorded the published findings from each study, and a third reviewer compared the two sets of data collection sheets and resolved any differences through discussion. Authors of the individual trials were contacted to verify data and obtain additional unpublished information.

Follow-Up: For the 56 trials for which follow-up data were available, the mean duration of follow-up was 62 days postoperatively.

Endpoints: All-cause mortality and morbidity (deep vein thrombosis, pulmo-nary embolism, myocardial infarction, transfusion requirements, pneumonia, other infections, respiratory depression, and renal failure).

RESULTS

- Overall mortality was reduced by one-third in patients allocated to neuraxial blockade (odds ratio = 0.70, confidence interval = 0.54–0.90, $P = 0.006$). Mortality was reduced overall whether neuraxial blockade was continued postoperatively or not.
- Of the 247 deaths within 30 days of randomization, a specific diagnosis was available for 162 (of these, 73 were due to pulmonary embolism, cardiac events, or stroke; 50 were due to infective causes; and 39 were due to other causes).
- There was limited power to assess subgroup effects, but proportional reduction in mortality did not differ by surgical group or blockade type (epidural or spinal) or in trials in which neuraxial blockade was combined with general anesthesia compared with trials in which neuraxial blockade was used alone.
- Neuraxial blockade reduced the odds of deep vein thrombosis by 44%, pulmonary embolism by 55%, transfusion requirements by 50%, pneumonia by 39%, and respiratory depression by 59% (all $P < 0.001$).
- There were reductions in myocardial infarction and renal failure, but the confidence intervals were compatible with both no effect and a halving of risk for myocardial infarction and both no effect and a two-thirds reduction of risk for renal failure.

Criticisms and Limitations: While the authors of this systematic review went to great lengths to obtain quality data, it is possible that some outcomes were missed. The confidence intervals were wide for several outcomes, including myocardial infarction and renal failure. None of the studies included in the analysis were individually powered to detect a clinically significant reduction in mortality from the use of neuraxial anesthesia, which may therefore be the principal reason that prior individual trials concluded that neuraxial blockade had no effect on mortality.

Other Relevant Studies and Information:

- A systematic review and meta-analysis of 125 trials published in 2014 examined whether adding epidural analgesia to general anesthesia decreased postoperative morbidity and mortality. Epidural analgesia significantly decreased the risk for morbidity (atrial fibrillation, supraventricular tachycardia, deep vein thrombosis, respiratory depression, atelectasis, pneumonia, ileus, and postoperative nausea and vomiting) as well as improved recovery of bowel function. However, technical failures occurred in 6.1% of patients, and epidural analgesia significantly increased the risk for arterial hypotension, pruritus, urinary retention, and motor blockade.[2]

- A systematic review published in 2016 of 14 randomized controlled trials compared paravertebral blockade with thoracic epidural blockade in adults undergoing elective thoracotomy and examined analgesic efficacy, the incidence of major and minor complications, length of hospital stay, and cost-effectiveness. Paravertebral blockade, compared with thoracic epidural blockade, reduced the risks for minor complications (hypotension, nausea and vomiting, pruritis, and urinary retention). Paravertebral blockade was as effective as thoracic epidural blockade in controlling acute pain. There was no difference in 30-day mortality, major complications, or length of hospital stay; data were insufficient on chronic pain and costs.[3]

Summary and Implications: This systematic review demonstrated that neuraxial blockade reduces morbidity and postoperative complications in a wide range of patients, independent of surgery type, choice of neuraxial technique, or use of general anesthesia.

CLINICAL CASE: EPIDURAL ANALGESIA

Case History

A 67-year-old woman presents for abdominal laparotomy for resection of an abdominal tumor. The patient has moderate chronic obstructive pulmonary disease and a history of nausea and vomiting with narcotic use. The patient is concerned about postoperative pain. How would neuraxial blockade be beneficial in this patient?

Suggested Answer

Epidural analgesia in addition to general anesthesia in this patient would be beneficial from a respiratory and nausea standpoint because neuraxial blockade has been shown to decrease postoperative morbidity such as respiratory depression and postoperative nausea and vomiting. If appropriate, epidural analgesia could be supplemented with multimodal, nonnarcotic analgesics such as acetaminophen or nonsteroidal anti-inflammatory drugs.

References

1. Rodgers A, Walker N, Schug S, et al. Reduction of postoperative mortality and morbidity with epidural or spinal anaesthesia: results from overview of randomised trials. *BMJ*. 2000 Dec 16;321(7275):1493.
2. Pöpping DM, Elia N, Van Aken HK, et al. Impact of epidural analgesia on mortality and morbidity after surgery: systematic review and meta-analysis of randomized controlled trials. *Ann Surg*. 2014 Jun;259(6):1056–67.
3. Yeung JH, Gates S, Naidu BV, Wilson MJ, Gao Smith F. Paravertebral block versus thoracic epidural for patients undergoing thoracotomy. *Cochrane Database Syst Rev*. 2016 Feb 21;2:CD009121.

43

Epidural Anesthesia and Analgesia in High-Risk Patients Undergoing Major Surgery

The improvement in analgesia, reduction in respiratory failure, and the low risk of serious adverse consequences suggest that many high-risk patients undergoing major intraabdominal surgery will receive substantial benefit from combined general and epidural anesthesia intraoperatively with continuing postoperative epidural analgesia.

—RIGG ET AL.[1]

Research Question: Do intraoperative epidural anesthesia and postoperative analgesia in high-risk patients presenting for major surgery decrease adverse outcomes compared with alternative analgesic regimens?

Funding: Australian and New Zealand College of Anaesthetists, the Health Department of Western Australia, and the National Health and Medical Research Council.

Year Study Began: 1995.

Year Study Published: 2002.

Study Location: 25 hospitals in six countries (Hong Kong, Malaysia, Australia, Saudi Arabia, Singapore, and Thailand).

Who Was Studied: High-risk patients undergoing elective, nonlaparoscopic abdominal or thoracic surgery (except for cardiac and pulmonary) lasting longer than 1 hour with one or more of the following characteristics preoperatively: morbid obesity, diabetes mellitus, chronic renal failure, respiratory insufficiency, major hepatocellular disease, recent cardiac disease (cardiac failure, myocardial infarction, or myocardial ischemia documented within previous 2 years) and age ≥75 years on day of surgery plus at least two significant risk factors (significant respiratory disease, cardiac dysrhythmia, hypertension, moderate obesity, frailty, myocardial infarction documented at any time).

Who Was Excluded: Patients <18 years of age, those undergoing surgery within 12 hours of admission, and those with contraindications to epidural placement (sepsis, infection at the epidural insertion site, impaired coagulation status, impaired mental status, or a neurologic disorder).

How Many Patients: 915.

Study Overview: See Figure 43.1 for an overview of the study's design.

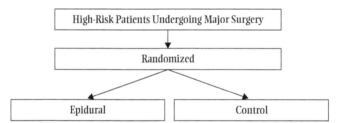

Figure 43.1 Summary of the study design.

Study Intervention: This randomized controlled trial provided participating centers with protocols for perioperative care addressing premedication, site of epidural placement, use of epidural local anesthetics and opioids intraoperatively and postoperatively, intraoperative monitoring, induction and maintenance of general anesthesia, replacement of blood and fluids, optimization of core temperature and cardiopulmonary function, extubation criteria, and immediate postoperative management. All patients underwent general anesthesia. The epidural group had an epidural placed before induction of anesthesia at a site selected by the attending anesthetist to match the planned incision with postoperative analgesia lasting for 72 hours consisting of a continuous infusion of bupivacaine or ropivacaine supplemented with meperidine or fentanyl. The control group received either a patient-controlled or physician-controlled opioid infusion for postoperative analgesia that was supplemented by rectal and oral nonsteroidal anti-inflammatory drugs, oral opioids, and acetaminophen.

Follow-Up: 30 days postoperatively.

Endpoints: Primary outcomes: postoperative death, respiratory failure, cardiovascular events, renal failure, gastrointestinal failure, hepatic failure, hematologic failure, inflammation/sepsis, and the combination of death or at least one endpoint. Secondary outcomes: intraoperative hemodynamics (maximum and minimum heart rate and systolic blood pressure) and postoperative pain assessed using a visual analog scale (VAS).

RESULTS

- A total of 27 patients were excluded after randomization because of cancellation of operation or ineligible procedure, leaving 888 patients (447 in the epidural group and 441 in the control group) included in the intension-to-treat analysis. Two or more study eligibility risk factors occurred in 33% of the control group vs. 26.5% of the epidural group ($P = 0.04$).
- Of the 447 epidural patients in the intention-to-treat analysis, 225 were fully compliant with protocol (breaches of protocol included epidural removal before leaving the operating room or before 72 hours postoperatively, insertion postoperatively, or inability to place catheter). Of the 441 patients assigned to the control group, 19 had epidural analgesia preoperatively or within 72 hours postoperatively.
- Epidural blockade was associated with significantly lower maximum heart rate and systolic blood pressure during surgery.
- Postoperative pain scores on the 10-cm VAS were significantly lower in the epidural group compared with the control group on the first postoperative day at rest and with coughing on postoperative days 1 to 3.
- Of the primary endpoints, there was significant reduction in the epidural group compared with the control group with regard to respiratory failure (number needed to treat = 15); respiratory failure occurred in 23% of epidural vs. 30% of control group patients ($P = 0.02$).
- There was no significant difference in mortality or the combined outcome of mortality and morbidity between the two study groups

(57.1% of patients in the epidural group vs. 60.7% of patients in the control group). An "as treated" analysis that reallocated control patients who received an epidural and epidural-group patients who did not receive an epidural yielded similar results.

Criticisms and Limitations: Treatment allocation could not be blinded. There was breech of study protocol in a large portion of patients because of the timing of epidural insertion or removal. If the true benefit associated with epidural use in high-risk patients is 3.6%, then the size of the study lacked power to detect this difference as statistically significant.

Other Relevant Studies and Information:
- A review of 15 randomized controlled studies comparing epidural analgesia to systemic opioid-based medications for elective open abdominal aortic surgery found epidural analgesia to provided better pain management and reduce the incidence of myocardial infarction, time to tracheal extubation, postoperative respiratory failure, gastrointestinal bleeding, and intensive care unit length of stay compared with systemic opioid-based drugs. There was no significant difference for postoperative mortality at 30 days.[2]

Summary and Implications: This multicenter, randomized trial demonstrated improved pain control and a reduction in postoperative respiratory complications with the use of an epidural for intraoperative anesthesia and postoperative analgesia in high-risk patients undergoing major surgery. A significant effect on overall complications or mortality was not demonstrated.

CLINICAL CASE: MAJOR ABDOMINAL SURGERY IN A HIGH-RISK PATIENT

Case History
A 67-year-old man presents for exploratory laparotomy for resection of a gastrointestinal tumor. The patient has chronic obstructive pulmonary disease and uses home oxygen occasionally. Additionally, he is obese (body mass index of 38) and has diabetes managed with oral medication. The patient

occasionally takes oxycodone at home for osteoarthritis pain, which limits his functional status. Given the patient's medical history and planned procedure, what should be the intraoperative and postoperative pain management plan?

Suggested Answer

This patient is at significant risk for postoperative cardiopulmonary complications. An epidural would be of benefit in the setting of multimodal analgesia to optimize the patient's pulmonary status postoperatively.

References

1. Rigg JR, Jamrozik K, Myles PS, et al. Epidural anaesthesia and analgesia and outcome of major surgery: a randomised trial. *Lancet.* 2002 Apr 13;359(9314):1276–82.
2. Guay J, Kopp S. Epidural pain relief versus systemic opioid-based pain relief for abdominal aortic surgery. Cochrane Database Syst Rev. 2016 Jan 5;1:CD005059.

44

Nerve Stimulator and Multiple Injection Technique for Upper and Lower Limb Blockade

Using the multiple injections technique with nerve stimulator provided successful nerve block in up to 94% of patients using volumes of local anesthetic less than those usually reported . . . the withdrawal and redirection of the stimulating needle was not associated with an increased incidence of nerve injury.

—FANELLI ET AL.[1]

Research Question: For peripheral nerve blocks performed using the multiple injection technique with a nerve stimulator, what are the failure rate, patient acceptance, effective volume of local anesthetic solution, and incidence of neurologic complications?

Funding: Italian Society of Anesthesia, Analgesia, and Intensive Care and by the IRCC H, San Raffaele, Milan, Italy.

Year Study Began: 1993.

Year Study Published: 1999.

Study Location: 28 hospitals in Italy.

Who Was Studied: All patients who consented for a peripheral nerve block for surgery involving either the upper or lower limb.

Who Was Excluded: Patients with a history of neuropathy or diabetes, those undergoing surgical procedures involving nervous structures, and those unable to consent.

How Many Patients: 3,996.

Study Overview: See Figure 44.1 for an overview of the study's design.

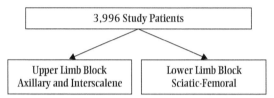

Figure 44.1 Summary of the study design.

Study Intervention: Standardized instructions for data collection and performance of nerve blocks were provided to anesthesiologists. Axillary, interscalene, or combined sciatic-femoral nerve blocks were performed with one of three available local anesthetic solutions using the multiple injection technique. Premedication consisted of oral diazepam or intramuscular (IM) droperidol. All blocks were performed with a short-beveled, Teflon-coated needle and a nerve stimulator with the frequency set at 2 Hz and stimulating current initially set to 1 mA and gradually decreased to <0.5 mA. Paresthesias were never intentionally sought; if unintentional paresthesia was elicited, no anesthetic was injected, the needle was withdrawn, and the procedure was re-peated. During block placement, proper needle placement was confirmed by appropriate muscular twitch responses. Recommended total doses of each type of local anesthetic were not exceeded. No routine sedation was given intraoperatively. The nerve block was considered unsuccessful if either a supplementary nerve block or general anesthesia was required to complete the surgery.

Follow-Up: 3 months.

Endpoints: Primary outcomes: failure rate, patient acceptance, effective volumes of local anesthetic solution, and incidence of neurologic complications. Secondary outcomes: use of vasoconstrictor, occurrence of unintentional paresthesia, adverse systemic local anesthetic reactions, duration of surgery, and duration and tourniquet inflation pressure.

RESULTS

- Of the 3,996 peripheral nerve blocks, 1,821 (46%) were brachial plexus blocks and 2,175 (54%) were combined sciatic-femoral blocks. For upper extremity blocks, 1,650 (42%) were axillary and 171 (4%) were interscalene.
- There were no cases of systemic adverse local anesthetic reactions. There was no association between the type of local anesthetic injected and neurologic dysfunction.
- The mean failure rate for all three nerve block groups was 7%.
- Patients receiving combined sciatic-femoral nerve blocks showed a worse acceptance of the procedure and reported more discomfort during block placement compared with axillary and interscalene blocks. Only 74% of patients would request the same anesthetic procedure if they underwent another surgery, mainly owing to discomfort during peripheral nerve block placement.
- Neurologic dysfunction developed in 69 (1.7%) of patients during the first month after surgery, with 68 patients recovering completely within 3 months. One patient required up to 25 weeks after surgery for neurologic recovery and demonstrated mild signs of peripheral nerve disease in the femoral nerve distribution on electrophysiologic evaluation performed 3 months after surgery.
- Unintentional paresthesia was elicited in 15% of patients during block placement (more often during brachial plexus blocks than combined sciatic-femoral blocks) but was not associated with postoperative neurologic complications.
- The incidence of neurologic dysfunction was highest in patients receiving interscalene blocks compared with axillary blocks ($P < 0.005$), but there was no difference between brachial plexus blocks and combined sciatic-femoral blocks.
- On univariate analysis, only type of nerve block and tourniquet inflation pressure were associated with the development of postoperative neurologic dysfunction. On multiple regression analysis, only tourniquet inflation pressure was associated with an increased risk for transient nerve injury (<400 mm Hg compared with >400 mm Hg; odds ratio = 2.9; 95% confidence interval = 1.6–5.4; $P < 0.001$).

Criticisms and Limitations: This study lacked a control group receiving either an "immobile needle" block technique or other technique used for needle location confirmation (such as ultrasound); thus, it is not possible to know how outcomes would have compared with other approaches. The number of muscular twitches elicited during block placement was not recorded and could not be correlated with outcomes. Neurologic function was evaluated only by physical examination, except for one patient who had neurologic dysfunction for >3 months and underwent electrophysiologic testing. Anesthesiology practitioners evaluating the patients postoperatively were not blinded.

Other Relevant Studies and Information:
- For axillary peripheral nerve blocks, nerve localization by nerve stimulation resulted in a greater success rate and a faster onset compared with paresthesia elicitation. The frequency of venous puncture was greater in the paresthesia group.[2]
- Paresthesias can occur without motor response from nerve stimulation, and a lack of motor response does not rule out the possibility of sensory nerve contact by the injection needle.[3]
- The use of ultrasound for needle location confirmation is now common practice. Studies examining the use of ultrasound during peripheral nerve block procedures have demonstrated reduced complication rates and improved quality, performance time, and time to block onset.[4]

Summary and Implications: Use of the multiple injection technique with a nerve stimulator during peripheral nerve block placement has a high success rate with a <2% incidence of transient neurologic complications. Elevated tourniquet inflation pressure was associated with an increased risk for transient nerve injury. However, only 74% of patients would request the same anesthetic procedure if they underwent another surgery, mainly owing to discomfort during peripheral nerve block placement.

CLINICAL CASE: PREOPERATIVE PERIPHERAL NERVE BLOCK

Case History
A 45-year-old woman presents for lower extremity surgery with preoperative combined sciatic-femoral peripheral nerve block. The patient is morbidly

obese and has obstructive sleep apnea. Although she has a low pain tolerance and fear of needles, she has consented to the block procedure. How should this patient's peripheral nerve block be performed given her body habitus and concerns regarding pain?

Suggested Answer

A successful peripheral nerve block in this patient would be ideal given her body habitus and likely airway concerns if deep sedation during the surgical procedure or postoperative narcotics are needed. This patient should be premedicated for her peripheral nerve block given her low pain tolerance, fear of needles, and need for two different skin punctures. Paresthesia elicitation should be avoided, which would increase discomfort. Needle location confirmation could be achieved with ultrasound, which may be of benefit given the patient's body habitus. A nerve stimulator would further aid nerve localization; however, it is possible to elicit paresthesia without eliciting a motor response.

References

1. Fanelli G, Casati A, Garancini P, Torri G. Nerve stimulator and multiple injection technique for upper and lower limb blockade: failure rate, patient acceptance, and neurologic complications. Study Group on Regional Anesthesia. *Anesth Analg.* 1999 Apr;88(4):847–52.
2. Sia S, Bartoli M, Lepri A, Marchini O, Ponsecchi P. Multiple-injection axillary brachial plexus block: a comparison of two methods of nerve localization-nerve stimulation versus paresthesia. *Anesth Analg.* 2000 Sep;91(3):647–51.
3. Urmey WF, Stanton J. Inability to consistently elicit a motor response following sensory paresthesia during interscalene block administration. *Anesthesiology.* 2002 Mar;96(3):552–4.
4. Walker KJ, McGrattan K, Aas-Eng K, Smith AF. Ultrasound guidance for peripheral nerve blockade. *Cochrane Database Syst Rev.* 2009 Oct 7;(4):CD006459.

Obstetric Anesthesiology

45

Neuraxial Analgesia Given Early in Labor

Neuraxial analgesia in early labor did not increase the rate of cesarean delivery, and it provided better analgesia and resulted in a shorter duration of labor than systemic analgesia.

—WONG ET AL.[1]

Research Question: What is the rate of cesarean delivery following neuraxial analgesia compared with systemic opioid analgesia administered in early labor?

Funding: Department of Anesthesiology, Feinberg School of Medicine, Northwestern University.

Year Study Began: 2000.

Year Study Published: 2005.

Study Location: Prentice Women's Hospital in Chicago, Illinois.

Who Was Studied: Healthy, nulliparous women with term, singleton pregnancies who presented in spontaneous labor or with spontaneous rupture of the membranes and desired neuraxial analgesia.

Who Was Excluded: Nonvertex presentation, scheduled induction of labor, any contraindication to opioid analgesia, and cervical dilation of 4 cm or greater.

How Many Patients: 750.

Study Overview: See Figure 45.1 for an overview of the study's design.

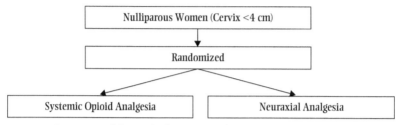

Figure 45.1 Summary of the study design.

Study Intervention: At the first request for analgesia, if cervical dilation was <4 cm, study participants were randomized to either systemic opioid analgesia (hydromorphone 1 mg intravenous [IV] and 1 mg intramuscular [IM]) or neuraxial analgesia (intrathecal fentanyl 25 mcg and epidural test dose). Epidural analgesia was initiated in the neuraxial group at the second request for analgesia and in the systemic opioid group at a cervical dilation of ≥4 cm or at the third request for analgesia. Thereafter, patient-controlled epidural analgesia was maintained in both groups until delivery. Study participates were asked to rate their pain according to an 11-point verbal rating score (in which 0 represents no pain and 10 represents the worst pain) at the first and second requests for analgesia. At the second request for analgesia, study participants were asked to rate their average pain with contractions since the start of the analgesic intervention as well as to rate their nausea and report any vomiting.

Follow-Up: Patients were followed until the time of delivery, including the assignment of neonatal Apgar scores.

Endpoints: Primary outcome: method of delivery (cesarean, instrumental, or spontaneous vaginal). Secondary outcomes: indication for cesarean delivery, method of vaginal delivery, quality of analgesia, use or nonuse of oxytocin, duration of labor, incidence of nonreassuring fetal status, neonatal outcome.

RESULTS

- There was no significant difference between the two study groups in the rate, indication for, or time to cesarean delivery. There was no significant difference between privately insured and publicly insured subjects or among different obstetric providers.

- On multivariate analysis, the method of providing analgesia was not a significant independent predictor of cesarean delivery.
- There was no significant difference in the rate of instrumental vaginal delivery.
- There was no significant difference in the percentages of subjects who received oxytocin. The maximum rate of oxytocin infusion was higher in the systemic analgesia group.
- There were no significant differences between the groups in the duration of the second stage of labor.
- The median times from the initiation of analgesic intervention to complete dilation (295 minutes vs. 385 minutes, $P < 0.001$) and to vaginal delivery (398 minutes vs. 479 minutes, $P < 0.001$) were significantly shorter after neuraxial analgesia than after systemic analgesia.
- Pain scores after the initial intervention were significantly lower with neuraxial than systemic analgesia (2 vs. 6 on a 1-to-10 scale, $P < 0.001$). The interval between the first and second requests for analgesia was significantly longer in the systemic analgesia group.
- The severity of nausea and the incidence of nausea and vomiting were lower in the neuraxial group.
- There was a higher incidence of prolonged and late decelerations in heart rate in the neuraxial group within 30 minutes after the initiation of analgesia, but there was no difference in the incidence of fetal heart rate tracings requiring an obstetric intervention.
- One-minute Apgar scores below 7 occurred significantly more frequently after systemic analgesia compared with neuraxial analgesia (24% vs. 16.7%, $P = 0.01$).

Criticisms and Limitations: The study included nulliparous women with singleton pregnancies in spontaneous labor or with spontaneous rupture of the membranes, and these results may not be applicable to other patient populations. Patients and care providers were not blinded to study group assignments. Epidural analgesia was not identical among all subjects. The study was not powered to detect a small difference between the two analgesic groups in the rate of cesarean delivery.

Other Relevant Studies and Information:

- This research paper was referenced by the American College of Obstetricians and Gynecologists (ACOG) 1 year later, writing that:

  ACOG reaffirms the opinion it published jointly with the American Society of Anesthesiologists, in which the following statement was articulated: "Labor causes severe pain for many women. There is no other circumstance where it is considered acceptable for an individual to experience untreated severe pain, amenable to safe intervention, while under a physician's care. In the absence of a medical contraindication, maternal request is a sufficient medical indication for pain relief during labor." The fear of unnecessary cesarean delivery should not influence the method of pain relief that women can choose during labor.[2]

Summary and Implications: The results of this randomized trial demonstrated that nulliparous women in spontaneous labor or with spontaneous rupture of the membranes who request analgesia early in labor can receive neuraxial analgesia at that time without adverse consequences. Compared with systemic opioid analgesia, neuraxial analgesia did not increase the risk for cesarean delivery and was associated with a lower rate of neonatal 1-minute Apgar scores below 7.

CLINICAL CASE: EPIDURAL ANALGESIA DURING LABOR

Case History
A 27-year-old, generally healthy, G1P0 woman presents for labor and birth. On examination, the patient is 4 cm dilated and requesting epidural analgesia. During the discussion of risks, benefits, and alternatives, the patient expresses concern that an epidural would prolong her labor or increase her risk for a cesarean delivery. How should these concerns be addressed?

Suggested Answer
It should be explained to the patient that epidural analgesia in early labor has not been shown to increase the rate of cesarean delivery. Regarding the duration of labor, epidural analgesia has been shown to shorten the duration of labor compared with systemic analgesia.

References

1. Wong CA, Scavone BM, Peaceman AM, et al. The risk of cesarean delivery with neuraxial analgesia given early versus late in labor. *N Engl J Med.* 2005 Feb 17;352(7):655–65.
2. Analgesia and Cesarean Delivery Rates. ACOG Committee Opinion No. 339. American College of Obstetricians and Gynecologists. *Obstet Gynecol.* 2006;107:1487–88.

46

Postdural Puncture Headache in Obstetrics: A Meta-analysis

[Postdural puncture headache] is a common complication for parturients undergoing neuraxial blockade.

—CHOI ET AL.[1]

Research Question: What are the frequency, onset, and duration of postdural puncture headache (PDPH) in the obstetric population after neuraxial blockade?

Funding: St. Joseph's Hospital Anesthesiologists' Research Fund.

Year Study Began: 1999.

Year Study Published: 2003.

Study Location: Three institutions in Canada and the United States.

Who Was Studied: Citations of obstetric populations undergoing neuraxial blockade that included extractable data on frequency, onset, and duration of PDPH.

Who Was Excluded: Citations that were abstracts or duplicate publications.

How Many Patients: 51 studies.

Study Overview: See Figure 46.1 for an overview of the study's design.

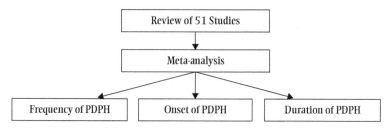

Figure 46.1 Summary of the study design.

Study Intervention: This meta-analysis combined prior obstetric research to extract information on the type of intervention (epidural, spinal, combined spinal and epidural [CSE]), needle design, number and frequency of accidental dural punctures (ADP) (if epidural), PDPH, and the onset and duration of PDPH from each citation by two independent reviewers.

Endpoints: Pooled estimates of frequency of ADP for epidural needles, frequencies of PDPH for epidural and spinal needles, onset of PDPH, and duration of PDPH.

RESULTS

- For epidurals, the pooled risk for ADP in obstetric patients was 1.5% (95% confidence interval [CI] = 1.5%–1.5%) during insertion for all epidural needles. After dural puncture occurred, the risk for developing a PDPH was 52.1% (95% CI = 51.4%–52.8%).
- For spinals, the risk for PDPH varied depending on the type of spinal needle and ranged from 1.5% to 11.2%. Whitacre atraumatic needles had lower PDPH risk compared with Quincke cutting needles of the same diameter (25-gauge: 2.2% vs. 6.3%, $P < 0.001$; 27-gauge: 1.7% vs. 2.9%, $P = 0.008$). The difference in PDPH risk between Sprotte and Quincke 24-gauge needles was not statistically significant.
- For CSE anesthesia, data were not pooled because of variation in the types of needles used.
- The onset of PDPH ranged from less than 1 day to 6 days after ADP during epidural insertion. For spinal needles, the onset of PDPH ranged from 1 to 7 days after dural puncture. The heterogeneity of data

presentation in the included studies prevented determination of median or mean times of onset for PDPH.

- Duration of PDPH ranged from 12 hours to 7 days.

Criticisms and Limitations: Studies in this meta-analysis varied with regard to duration of patient follow-up, prophylactic and therapeutic interventions for PDPH, and sample size for each type of needle. In each case, prospective studies suggested higher risks than retrospective studies, signifying possible underreporting in retrospective studies. The severity of PDPH was not characterized in this analysis, and pooled estimates were not adjusted for operator skill.

Other Relevant Studies and Information:

- A retrospective analysis[2] of 17,198 parturients who underwent neuraxial blockade between 1997 and 2006 found the incidence of PDPH to be similar after puncture with needle and catheter, after epidural and CSE techniques, after 27-gauge and 29-gauge pencil-point spinal needles, and after spinal and epidural catheter insertion (61% vs. 52%; $P > 0.05$). All headaches presented within 72 hours. The ADP rate was similar among residents and staff, but residents had "gained extensive experience performing epidural and CSE anaesthesia before their rotation to the labour and delivery ward."
- A retrospective analysis[3] of 29,749 parturients who underwent neuraxial blockade between 1997 and 2013 found the incidence of PDPH to be significantly reduced when the epidural catheter was inserted intrathecally for at least 24 hours compared with when the catheter was resited epidurally after witnessed ADP (42% vs. 62%; $P = 0.04$).
- A retrospective analysis[4] of 238 ADPs between 2002 and 2010 found the insertion of an intrathecal catheter following accidental dural puncture to significantly decrease the incidence of PDPH compared with epidural catheter insertion at a different level (37% vs. 54%; $P = 0.03$). The need for an epidural blood patch following intrathecal catheter insertion was reduced, but the difference did not reach statistical significance.

Summary and Implications: This meta-analysis found that PDPH is a frequent complication, with an estimated incidence of 1.5% for epidurals and 52.1% when dural puncture occurs. For spinals, the risk for PDPH varied depending on the type of spinal needle and ranged from 1.5% to 11.2%. The conclusions of this meta-analysis are consistent with prior recommendations that smallest diameter, atraumatic needles be used for spinal analgesia or anesthesia.

CLINICAL CASE: EPIDURAL PLACEMENT FOR LABOR ANALGESIA

Case History

A 22-year-old woman, G1P0, is in active labor and requests epidural analgesia. The patient is healthy, has a body mass index of 29, does not have contraindications to neuraxial blockade, and is 5 cm dilated. What is important to discuss with the patient regarding the risks for ADP and PDPH?

Suggested Answer

A discussion of risks, benefits, and alternatives should precede the procedure. Regarding ADP during epidural placement, the risk is relatively small. It is important to mention that if dural puncture occurs, the risk for developing a PDPH is about 50%. Recent studies indicate that threading an epidural catheter into the intrathecal space in the event of a witnessed ADP reduces the incidence of PDPH. Possible therapy options, including the need for an epidural blood patch, should be discussed.

References

1. Choi PT, Galinski SE, Takeuchi L, Lucas S, Tamayo C, Jadad AR. PDPH is a common complication of neuraxial blockade in parturients: a meta-analysis of obstetrical studies. *Can J Anaesth.* 2003 May;50(5):460–9.
2. Van de Velde M, Schepers R, Berends N, Vandermeersch E, De Buck F. Ten years of experience with accidental dural puncture and post-dural puncture headache in a tertiary obstetric anaesthesia department. *Int J Obstet Anesth.* 2008 Oct;17(4):329–35.
3. Verstraete S, Walters MA, Devroe S, Roofthooft E, Van de Velde M. Lower incidence of post-dural puncture headache with spinal catheterization after accidental dural puncture in obstetric patients. *Acta Anaesthesiol Scand.* 2014 Nov;58(10):1233–39.
4. Kaddoum R, Motlani F, Kaddoum RN, Srirajakalidindi A, Gupta D, Soskin V. Accidental dural puncture, postdural puncture headache, intrathecal catheters, and epidural blood patch: revisiting the old nemesis. *J Anesth.* 2014 Aug;28(4):628–30.

Pediatric Anesthesiology

47

Parental Presence During Induction vs. Sedative Premedication

Oral midazolam is more effective than either parental presence or no intervention for managing a child's and parent's anxiety during the preoperative period.

—KAIN ET AL.[1]

Research Question: Is a pharmacologic intervention (midazolam premedication) or a behavioral intervention (parental presence) more effective in reducing
anxiety of children undergoing surgery?

Funding: Roche Pharmaceuticals and the National Institutes of Health.

Year Study Began: 1996.

Year Study Published: 1998.

Study Location: Yale-New Haven Children's Hospital, New Haven, Connecticut.

Who Was Studied: Children 2 to 8 years of age with an American Society of
Anesthesiologists (ASA) physical status I or II undergoing elective outpatient
surgery under general anesthesia.

Who Was Excluded: Children with any history of chronic illness, prematurity, or developmental delay and children of parents who insisted on a particular study group.

How Many Patients: 88.

Study Overview: See Figure 47.1 for an overview of the study's design.

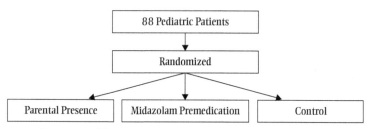

Figure 47.1 Summary of the study design.

Study Intervention: In this randomized controlled study, participants were recruited either the night before surgery or 2–7 days before surgery while undergoing a preoperative preparation program. Subjects were randomized into three groups: parental presence, midazolam premedication, or control. For the parental presence group, standardized instructions were given, and one parent accompanied the child into the operating room and stayed for induction of anesthesia. For the premedication group, 0.5 mg/kg oral midazolam mixed in 10 mg/kg acetaminophen syrup was administered at least 20 minutes before the procedure. For the control group, children went into the operating room without premedication or parental presence. All inductions were performed by a group of six anesthesiologists. A total of eight behavioral tools were used in this study: four were completed by the parent, three by an observer, and one by the child. A psychologist functioned as the assessor and administered the various observational tools in the preoperative holding area, on separation from the parent, on entrance to the operating room, and during induction of anesthesia. After the procedure, parents were asked to rate their satisfaction with nursing, anesthesia, and overall care. Two weeks after surgery, parents were contacted for a Posthospitalization Behavior Questionnaire.

Follow-Up: 2 weeks postoperatively.

Endpoints: Primary endpoint: anxiety of the child during the perioperative period. Secondary endpoints: anxiety of the parent, compliance of the child, various recovery measures (e.g., pain, nausea and vomiting), and parental satisfaction.

RESULTS

- Baseline characteristics were similar in the study groups with regard to age, gender, temperament, coping styles, and parental trait anxiety. In the preoperative holding area, there were no differences in the child's anxiety among the study groups.
- At the time of separation from parents, patients in the midazolam premedication group exhibited significantly less anxiety compared with the parental-presence and control groups ($P < 0.02$).
- At entrance to the operating room and application of the anesthesia mask, the midazolam premedication group was significantly less anxious than the parental-presence and control groups.
- Child compliance with induction was poor (defined by a score >6 on the Induction Compliance Checklist) in more patients in the control group than in the parental-presence and midazolam premedication groups (25% vs. 17% vs. 0%, $P = 0.013$).
- There were no significant differences among the three groups for induction times, rates of nausea or vomiting, time to recovery, incidence of postoperative excitement, or negative behavioral changes reported 2 weeks after surgery.
- Parental anxiety after separation was lower in the midazolam premedication group compared with the parental-presence and control groups ($P = 0.048$).
- Parent satisfaction with care was very high in all three study groups.

Criticisms and Limitations: The findings of this study may not be generalizable to anesthesia practices that selectively offer parental presence based on the personality characteristics of each child and parent. Blinding of the observer rating the child at separation, on arrival to the operating room, and during induction was not possible for the parental-presence group. The assessment instrument used to determine parent satisfaction may not have been sensitive enough to capture differences among the three study groups.

Other Relevant Studies and Information:

- A review[2] published in 2015 of 28 trials of nonpharmacologic interventions during induction of anesthesia in children found that parental presence during induction does not diminish their child's anxiety.

- A number of drug regimens have been studied for premedication in children undergoing anesthesia (e.g., midazolam, ketamine, clonidine, and dexmedetomidine).[3,4]
- A 2012 study[5] comparing intranasal dexmedetomidine and midazolam premedication found both drugs to be equally effective in decreasing anxiety on separation from parents. Midazolam was superior in providing satisfactory conditions during mask induction ($P < 0.01$), but the number of patients who required postoperative analgesia was higher in the midazolam group ($P = 0.045$).

Summary and Implications: This randomized controlled trial demonstrated that premedication with oral midazolam was more effective at reducing pre-operative anxiety in both children and parents than parental presence during induction. Furthermore, premedicated children were more compliant with induction.

CLINICAL CASE: PREOPERATIVE ANXIETY

Case History

A generally healthy, 6-year-old boy presents for outpatient orthopedic surgery. The patient has had two prior anesthetics for dental procedures at another institution, which the parents describe as "stressful" and "traumatic" because of separation anxiety. Premedication was not offered during prior anesthetics. How should this patient be managed in order to minimize preoperative anxiety and promote compliance with induction?

Suggested Answer

Given the description of prior anesthetic experiences, this patient would benefit from sedative premedication before induction. A number of premedication regimens could be chosen. Given that the surgery is orthopedic and likely to be painful during recovery, midazolam in acetaminophen syrup or intranasal dexmedetomidine would offer additional analgesic benefits. If parental presence is requested and deemed to be appropriate, the parent accompanying the patient into the operating room should receive instructions and information regarding the induction process.

References

1. Kain ZN, Mayes LC, Wang SM, Caramico LA, Hofstadter MB. Parental presence during induction of anesthesia versus sedative premedication: which intervention is more effective? *Anesthesiology.* 1998 Nov;89(5):1147–56; discussion 9A-10A.

2. Manyande A, Cyna AM, Yip P, Chooi C, Middleton P. Non-pharmacological interventions for assisting the induction of anaesthesia in children. *Cochrane Database Syst Rev.* 2015 Jul 14;7:CD006447.

3. Mitra S, Kazal S, Anand LK. Intranasal clonidine vs. midazolam as premedication in children: a randomized controlled trial. *Indian Pediatr.* 2014 Feb;51(2):113–18.

4. Darlong V, Shende D, Subramanyam MS, Sunder R, Naik A. Oral ketamine or midazolam or low dose combination for premedication in children. *Anaesth Intensive Care.* 2004 Apr;32(2):246–49.

5. Akin A, Bayram A, Esmaoglu A, et al. Dexmedetomidine vs midazolam for premedication of pediatric patients undergoing anesthesia. *Paediatr Anaesth.* 2012 Sep;22(9):871–76.

48

Perioperative Pediatric Morbidity and Mortality

Overall, about 40% of the children experienced at least one problem, whether in the intraoperative, recovery-room, or the later postoperative period.

—COHEN ET AL.[1]

Research Question: What are the rates of perioperative adverse events among children of different ages?

Funding: National Health Research Development Program

Year Study Published: 1990.

Study Location: Winnipeg Children's Hospital, University of Manitoba, Canada.

Who Was Studied: Perioperative pediatric anesthesia data from 1982 to 1987 for patients up to 16 years of age for all surgical procedures.

How Many Patients: 29,220 anesthetics.

Study Overview: See Figure 48.1 for an overview of the study's design.

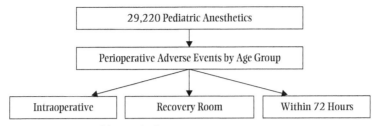

Figure 48.1 Summary of the study design.

Study Intervention: This study used data from 29,220 anesthetics collected from 1982 to 1987 and analyzed the rate of perioperative adverse events for children in five age groups: younger than 1 month, 1–12 months, 1–5 years, 6–10 years, and 11–16 years. The pediatric anesthesiologist who cared for each patient completed a check-off form for each case. A designated reviewer examined all forms and hospital charts to ascertain adverse effects in the intraoperative, recovery room, and postoperative periods. For inpatients, when possible, children and parents were interviewed to assess level of satisfaction and postoperative concerns. The check-off form was returned to the attending anesthesiologist for final review before processing; follow-up information was conducted simultaneously with billing requirements, leading to excellent compliance. Consistent definitions of study variables were used. An audit was conducted by reviewing and comparing 140 random database records with hospital charts; the information in the database regarding perioperative events was found to be coded reliably. Data were grouped into three time periods: 1982–83, 1984–85, and 1986–87.

Follow-Up: 72 hours postoperatively.

Endpoints: Intraoperative and recovery room events: arrhythmia, hypotension, hypothermia, laryngospasm, bronchospasm, drug incidents, and excessive bleeding. Postoperative events: muscular pain, dental injury, positional injury, eye injury, respiratory and cardiovascular events, hyperthermia, hepatic or renal abnormalities, arterial line complications (excessive bruising or loss of pulse), awareness, and surgical events (excessive bleeding, return to operating room).

RESULTS

- Most patients had no coexisting medical conditions (74%) and were classified as American Society of Anesthesiologists (ASA) physical status I or II (95%). Most cases were elective (89%) and inpatient (55%) and lasted less than 1 hour (52%). The main surgical categories were eye/ear-nose-throat (ENT) and musculoskeletal. Most cases used blood pressure, electrocardiogram, and a precordial/esophageal stethoscope for monitoring. Nitrous oxide was used in 96% of cases, and halothane was used in 91% of cases.

- Neonates had the highest age-specific rates for intracranial, intra-abdominal, or major vascular/cardiac procedures and were more likely to be ASA physical status III to V.
- Approximately 9% of cases had at least one intraoperative event. Neonates had the highest intraoperative rates of mortality and adverse events (most commonly respiratory). Infants 1–12 months of age had the fewest intraoperative events. For children 1–10 years of age, arrhythmia was the most frequent intraoperative event.
- In the recovery room, neonates had the highest rates of cardiac arrest and adverse events, with respiratory events and temperature changes being the most frequent. For infants, the rate of recovery room complications was low and most frequently associated with the respiratory system. Children 1–5 years of age and adolescents had a high incidence of respiratory events. The adolescent group also demonstrated high rates of vomiting, with an incidence of approximately 30%.
- In 22,760 cases (78% of all anesthetics), review was conducted of the 72-hour postoperative period. For neonates, 62% had no adverse postoperative events, compared with 81% for infants and 59% for older children. During this period, neonates had the greatest amount of major postoperative events (defined as being life-threatening or with potential lasting morbidity). For neonates, the most common postoperative events were respiratory and cardiovascular. For infants, vomiting, respiratory, and temperature events were most common. For older children, nausea and vomiting were most common. Older children experienced more sore throats, headaches, and muscle pain.
- Despite the number of perioperative adverse events, there was little parental dissatisfaction with the anesthetic experience (approximately four per 10,000 anesthetics).
- Overall, approximately 40% of children experienced at least one perioperative adverse event. Over the 6 years of the study, there was a decrease in the rate of postoperative events.

Criticisms and Limitations: There was no attempt to distinguish between adverse events attributable to the surgical procedure vs. the anesthetic. Older children had higher rates of certain postoperative events (sore throat, headaches, and muscle aches), possibly because younger children are unable to express these symptoms. Whether an event was deemed important to include was subject to the interpretation of the individual completing the form; it is possible that minor events may have been underreported. Neonatal patients were routinely nursed in the neonatal intensive care unit, where greater level of care and observation may result in enhanced detection of perioperative events. The form used for data collection was created in the 1970s, thereby possibly not reflecting advances in knowledge, monitoring, or therapeutics. The high incidence of arrhythmias was likely secondary to halothane, which is no longer used routinely. Intraoperative monitoring during the time of the study did not include routine use of pulse oximetry or capnography. Postoperative vomiting rates were high, but patients did not receive antiemetics and were undergoing procedures now known to be associated with a high risk for postoperative nausea and vomiting.

Other Relevant Studies and Information:

- A more recent prospective study[2] analyzed 24,165 anesthetics and reported 724 adverse events (3%) during anesthesia and 1,105 adverse events (5%) in the postanesthesia care unit (PACU). Respiratory events represented 53% of intraoperative events and were more frequent in infants, ENT surgery, in children in whom the trachea was intubated, and in children with an ASA physical status III to V. Cardiac events accounted for 12.5% of intraoperative events and were mainly observed in children with an ASA physical status III to V. In the PACU, vomiting was the most frequent adverse event, particularly in older children and after ENT surgery.
- An analysis of the ASA Closed Claims Project in 1993[3] showed a higher proportion of closed pediatric malpractice claims to be related to respiratory events compared with adult claims (43% vs. 30% in adult claims; $P \leq 0.01$).
- The Pediatric Perioperative Cardiac Arrest (POCA) Registry[4] analysis of 289 cases from 1994 to 1997 found 150 of the arrests (52%) to be related to anesthesia, yielding an incidence of cardiac arrest of 1.4 ± 0.45 (mean ± SD) per 10,000 instances of anesthesia and a mortality rate of 26%. Anesthesia-related cardiac arrest occurred most often in patients with severe underlying disease and in patients younger than 1 year.
- Un update published by POCA in 2007[5] reviewed cases from 1998 to 2004 and found 193 arrests (49%) to be related to anesthesia. Cardiovascular causes were the most common (41%), with

hypovolemia from blood loss and hyperkalemia from transfusion the most common identifiable causes. Among respiratory causes of arrest (27%), airway obstruction from laryngospasm was the most common cause.

Summary and Implications: This was a large study that provided estimates of the rates for adverse perioperative events among children. It showed that almost half of children experience some type of perioperative complications.

CLINICAL CASE: PEDIATRIC PERIOPERATIVE COMPLICATIONS

Case History

A 16-year-old girl with appendicitis presents for laparoscopic appendectomy. During the preoperative evaluation, the parents ask about risks of anesthesia and rates of perioperative complications.

Suggested Answer

Given the patient's age and procedure, the likelihood of postoperative events such as nausea and vomiting and sore throat from the endotracheal tube should be explained. A discussion of rare complications such as cardiopulmonary events should be included when obtaining informed consent.

References

1. Cohen MM, Cameron CB, Duncan PG. Pediatric anesthesia morbidity and mortality in the perioperative period. *Anesth Analg.* 1990 Feb;70(2):160–67.
2. Murat I, Constant I, Maud'huy H. Perioperative anaesthetic morbidity in children: a database of 24,165 anaesthetics over a 30-month period. *Paediatr Anaesth.* 2004 Feb;14(2):158–66.
3. Morray JP, Geiduschek JM, Caplan RA, Posner KL, Gild WM, Cheney FW. A comparison of pediatric and adult anesthesia closed malpractice claims. *Anesthesiology.* 1993 Mar;78(3):461–67.
4. Morray JP, Geiduschek JM, Ramamoorthy C, et al. Anesthesia-related cardiac arrest in children: initial findings of the Pediatric Perioperative Cardiac Arrest (POCA) Registry. *Anesthesiology.* 2000 Jul;93(1):6–14.
5. Bhananker SM, Ramamoorthy C, Geiduschek JM, et al. Anesthesia-related cardiac arrest in children: update from the Pediatric Perioperative Cardiac Arrest Registry. *Anesth Analg.* 2007 Aug;105(2):344–50.

49

CRIES: A Neonatal Postoperative Pain Measurement Score

We have demonstrated that the CRIES score is a valid, reliable, highly acceptable tool which is easy to remember and easy to use.

—KRECHEL ET AL.[1]

Research Question: Is the CRIES score a valid and reliable method for assessing neonatal postoperative pain?

Year Study Published: 1995.

Study Location: University of Missouri-Columbia in Columbia, Missouri.

Who Was Studied: Infants admitted to the neonatal intensive care unit or to the pediatric intensive care unit following surgery.

How Many Patients: 24.

Study Overview: See Figure 49.1 for an overview of the study's design.

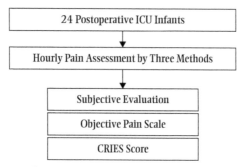

Figure 49.1 Summary of the study design.

Study Intervention: In the postoperative period, infants in the intensive care unit (ICU) were assessed hourly by two nurses using three methods: a subjective evaluation, the Objective Pain Scale (OPS), and the CRIES score. The subjective evaluation was based on the nurse's belief of whether or not the infant was in pain. The OPS was developed and validated in preverbal children and evaluates movement, agitation, body language, crying, and blood pressure. The CRIES score (Table 49.1) combined physiologic and behavioral parameters often associated with pain in neonates. Following each hourly assessment by two nurses, the results were shown to a third nurse who was designated as the consistent evaluator. A yes on the subjective evaluation or a score greater than six on either the OPS or CRIES was taken as an indication to administer analgesia as ordered. To test discriminant validity, OPS and CRIES scores at the time of analgesic administration and for the hour immediately following were extracted from the data and analyzed.

Table 49.1. CRIES SCORE*

Variable	Score of 0	Score of 1	Score of 2
Crying	No	High-pitched	Inconsolable
Requires oxygen for saturation >95%	No	<30%	>30%
Increased vital signs	HR and BP ≤ preop	HR or BP ↑ <20% of preop	HR or BP ↑ >20% of preop
Expression	None	Grimace	Grimace/grunt
Sleeplessness	No	Wakes at frequent intervals	Constantly awake

*Neonatal pain assessment tool developed at the University of Missouri-Columbia. Copyright S. Krechel, MD and J. Bildner, RNC, CNS.
BP = blood pressure; *HR* = heart rate.

Follow-Up: Up to 72 hours postoperatively.

Endpoints: Validity and reliability of CRIES score compared with subjective assessment and OPS. Nursing preference for CRIES vs. OPS.

RESULTS

- Patients ranged from 32 to 60 weeks gestational age (mean, 44 weeks) and were admitted to the ICU following various surgical procedures (e.g., neurosurgical, gastrointestinal, and cardiovascular). The period of assessment depended on the surgical procedure and ranged between 24 and 72 hours postoperatively. A total of 1,382 observations were made.
- The Spearman rank correlation coefficient is a nonparametric measure of statistical dependence between two variables and was found to be 0.73 between the OPS and CRIES scores $(P < 0.0001, n = 1,382)$.
- When the subjective assessment indicated the presence of pain, the median score on both OPS and CRIES was 4; when the subjective assessment indicated an absence of pain, the median score on both OPS and CRIES was 0. The Spearman correlation coefficient between the subjective report and a measurement using OPS or CRIES was 0.49 $(P < 0.0001, n > 1,300$ for both).
- Both OPS and CRIES demonstrated discriminant validity: with analgesic administration, the mean postmedication decline was 3.4 units for OPS $(P < 0.0001, n = 77)$ and 3 units for CRIES $(P < 0.0001, n = 74)$.
- Nurse pairs showed agreement on subjective evaluation 94% of the time. The Spearman correlation coefficient between raters showed reasonable agreement for both OPS $(r = 0.73, P < 0.0001, n = 659)$ and CRIES $(r = 0.72, P < 0.0001, n = 680)$.
- Of the nurses participating in this study, 73% indicated a preference for CRIES, 24% preferred OPS, and 3% preferred none.

Criticisms and Limitations: CRIES was validated against subjective assessment and OPS; however, these are also subjective measures. The CRIES score may not be appropriate for patients younger than 32 weeks gestational age, and the score cannot fully assess patients who are intubated, sedated, or paralyzed. The statistical analysis methods used in this study assume independent observations, but this condition was not strictly met because the nurse pairs contributed multiple observations.

Other Relevant Studies and Information:

- A 2006[2] comparison of postoperative pain scales in neonates prospectively cross-validated three pain scales: CRIES, Children's and Infants' Postoperative Pain Scale (CHIPPS), and the Neonatal Infant Pain Scale (NIPS) in terms of validity, reliability, and practicality. CRIES, CHIPPS, and NIPS were all valid and reliable. NIPS did not require calculating the change in vital signs and was therefore a more practical scale in a busy clinical setting.
- A study[3] published in 2011 compared assessment tools for evaluating pain in 81 full-term, critically ill neonates following cardiac surgery during the first 48 hours postoperatively. The following indices were measured: heart rate, mean arterial blood pressure, heart rate variability, urinary and plasma cortisol, and four composite pain measurement scales: CHIPPS, CRIES, COMFORT,[4] and Premature Infant Pain Profile (PIPP). The COMFORT score performed best, with both behavioral and physiologic components providing significant contributions.

Summary and Implications: Regular pain assessment and treatment in the neonatal population is important postoperatively. The CRIES scale was designed to measure pain in the neonatal population, and this study demonstrated CRIES to be a valid and reliable assessment tool for identifying postsurgical pain in neonates. Multiple pain assessment tools, including CRIES, are available for use in neonatal patients and in patient populations who are otherwise unable to verbalize discomfort.

CLINICAL CASE: NEONATAL POSTOPERATIVE ASSESSMENT

Case History

A neonatal patient of 44 weeks gestational age is admitted to the ICU postoperatively after pyloromyotomy. On one of the hourly pain assessments using the CRIES score, the baby is found to have a high-pitched cry, an increase in heart rate above 20% from the preoperative baseline, occasional grimacing, and sleeplessness for the duration of the prior hour. Based on these findings, what is the CRIES score, and should analgesics be administered?

Suggested Answer

Given the examination findings, the CRIES score would be tabulated as follows: 1 point for crying, 2 points for increased vital signs, 1 point for facial expression, 2 points for sleeplessness. Given a total score of 6, the neonate is likely in pain, and analgesics should be administered. A CRIES score of 4 or greater suggests that analgesics should be administered.

References

1. Krechel SW, Bildner J. CRIES: a new neonatal postoperative pain measurement score. Initial testing of validity and reliability. *Paediatr Anaesth.* 1995;5(1):53–61.
2. Suraseranivongse S, Kaosaard R, Intakong P, et al. A comparison of postoperative pain scales in neonates. *Br J Anaesth.* 2006 Oct;97(4):540–44.
3. Franck LS, Ridout D, Howard R, Peters J, Honour JW. A comparison of pain measures in newborn infants after cardiac surgery. *Pain.* 2011 Aug;152(8):1758–65.
4. Ambuel B, Hamlett KW, Marx CM, Blumer JL. Assessing distress in pediatric intensive care environments: the COMFORT scale. *J Pediatr Psychol.* 1992 Feb;17(1):95–109.

50

Emergence Agitation After Sevoflurane vs. Propofol in Pediatrics

In preschool children undergoing a minor procedure, the use of sevoflurane as a maintenance anesthetic causes a greater incidence of emergence agitation compared with propofol.

—Uezono et al.[1]

Research Question: Does maintenance of anesthesia with propofol after sevoflurane induction reduce the incidence of emergence agitation compared with continuing sevoflurane for maintenance?

Year Study Published: 2000.

Study Location: Department of Anesthesiology, Teikyo University and Ichihara Hospital, Chiba, Japan.

Who Was Studied: Pediatric patients 1 to 5 years of age diagnosed with retinoblastoma requiring routine eye examination under general anesthesia on a regular basis. Participants were American Society of Anesthesiologists (ASA) physical status I or II, they had prior procedures with inhalational anesthetics, and none had received prior propofol-based anesthesia.

Who Was Excluded: Patients who had a history of neurologic disorder or had undergone a series of radiation therapy requiring daily general anesthesia.

How Many Patients: 16.

Study Overview: See Figure 50.1 for an overview of the study's design.

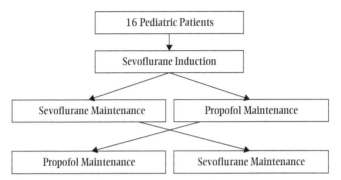

Figure 50.1 Summary of the study design.

Study Intervention: In this randomized, single-blinded, two-period, cross-over study, 16 pediatric patients underwent repeat eye examinations under general anesthesia. Oral midazolam 0.5 mg/kg was administered 30 minutes before induction with inhaled 5% sevoflurane in 95% oxygen. Patients were randomly assigned to one of two groups for maintenance—one group (eight patients) received sevoflurane for maintenance, with end-tidal concentrations of sevoflurane between 2% and 4%; the second group (eight patients) receive a 2-mg/kg bolus followed by a continuous infusion of 100 to 400 mcg/kg/min of propofol. Maintenance anesthetic doses were titrated to maintain heart rate and blood pressure within 20% of preinduction values. For the second procedure performed several months later, the alternative maintenance anesthetic was used under the same protocol. No opioids were administered intraoperatively. An anesthesiologist blinded to the type of maintenance anesthetic received assessed recovery immediately after the end of the procedure and in the postanesthesia care unit (PACU).

Follow-Up: At end of procedure and during PACU stay.

Endpoints: Primary outcome: presence or absence and duration of emergence agitation in the PACU (defined as inconsolable crying, combative behavior, or thrashing). Secondary outcomes: time from end of surgery to tracheal extubation, spontaneous eye opening, first oral intake, duration of PACU stay, incidence of emesis in the first 24 hours, the need for additional medications for pain relief, satisfaction of mothers with their child's anesthetic.

RESULTS

- Patients were seven boys and nine girls, ages 26 ± 15 months and weighing 14 ± 6 kg (mean $\pm$ SD, respectively). Anesthesia and surgery times were similar for the two groups. Rectal acetaminophen was administered to all patients after induction; no patients required additional medication for pain in the PACU or on the ward.
- The sevoflurane group experienced a faster recovery based on time to spontaneous eye opening ($P < 0.05$) and duration of PACU stay ($P < 0.01$), but these differences were clinically insignificant. See Table 50.1 for results.
- The incidence of emergence agitation occurred in six of 16 patients (38%) after sevoflurane maintenance compared with none after propofol maintenance ($P < 0.05$).
- For the six patients who developed emergence agitation after sevoflurane maintenance, the median duration of agitation was 8 minutes (range, 4–12 minutes). The agitation resolved without pharmacologic intervention and did not cause any cardiopulmonary compromise.
- After the 32 general anesthetics delivered, two episodes of postoperative emesis were recorded on the ward, both of which occurred after sevoflurane maintenance.
- Mothers of patients interviewed on the first postoperative morning rated the anesthesia experience as more favorable after propofol maintenance compared with sevoflurane maintenance ($P < 0.05$). Five of six parents whose children experienced emergence agitation after sevoflurane anesthesia expressed a preference for the propofol maintenance technique.

Table 50.1. SUMMARY OF KEY FINDINGS*

Recovery Characteristics	Propofol ($N = 16$)	Sevoflurane ($N = 16$)
Time to extubation (min)	16 ± 7	13 ± 4
Time to eye opening (min)	32 ± 16	$19 \pm 8^{\ddagger}$
Duration of PACU stay (min)	43 ± 10	$29 \pm 6^{\S}$

Recovery Characteristics	Propofol (N = 16)	Sevoflurane (N = 16)
Time to first oral intake (min)	139 ± 71	167 ± 79
Total incidence of agitation (%)	0 (0)	6 (38)[‡]
Parent satisfaction score[+]	5 (1)	4 (1.3)[‡]

*Values are mean ± SD except where indicated.
[+]Parent satisfaction score is reported as median (range) on scale of 1 = unsatisfied to 5 = highly satisfied.
[‡]$P < 0.05$.
[§]$P < 0.01$.

Criticisms and Limitations: Similar depths of anesthesia during maintenance with sevoflurane and propofol cannot be guaranteed. Parents were not allowed in the PACU, were unaware of duration of PACU stay, and did not witness episodes of emergence agitation; the differences in parent satisfaction would have likely been greater had parents witnessed the PACU portion of recovery. The procedure in this study was minimally invasive and nonpainful; pain may be a significant contributor to the occurrence of emergence agitation, limiting the applicability of the results of this study.

Other Relevant Studies and Information:

- Similarly to the results of this study, propofol has been demonstrated to reduce the incidence of emergence agitation in children in numerous studies.[2-6]
- Differing definitions of emergence delirium and agitation are used by various studies due to the heterogeneity of clinical presentations.[7,8]

Summary and Implications: In preschool children undergoing noninvasive, repeat eye examinations under general anesthesia, emergence agitation occurred more frequently after maintenance with sevoflurane compared with propofol. Sevoflurane maintenance resulted in statistically faster recovery times but lower parent satisfaction scores.

CLINICAL CASE: EMERGENCE AGITATION

Case History
A 4-year-old girl with a history of retinoblastoma presents for outpatient eye examination under general anesthesia. The patient has had multiple prior

anesthetics, after several of which she exhibited emergence agitation in the PACU. The patient's parents are concerned about recovery in the PACU and ask whether a certain type of anesthetic is known to decrease the incidence of emergence agitation.

Suggested Answer

Multiple studies link the use of sevoflurane maintenance with emergence agitation. Prior anesthetic records should be reviewed. Multiple agents have been demonstrated to decrease the incidence of emergence agitation, including propofol, alpha-2 agonists (dexmedetomidine, clonidine), opioids, and ketamine.[9] Given that this is a minimally invasive, nonpainful procedure, the type of anesthetic agent used should be weighed against speed of recovery and side effects. Sevoflurane should be avoided for maintenance, if possible.

References

1. Uezono S, Goto T, Terui K, et al. Emergence agitation after sevoflurane versus propofol in pediatric patients. *Anesth Analg.* 2000 Sep;91(3):563–66.
2. Picard V, Dumont L, Pellegrini M. Quality of recovery in children: sevoflurane versus propofol. *Acta Anaesthesiol Scand.* 2000 Mar;44(3):307–10.
3. Cohen IT, Finkel JC, Hannallah RS, Hummer KA, Patel KM. Rapid emergence does not explain agitation following sevoflurane anaesthesia in infants and children: a comparison with propofol. *Paediatr Anaesth.* 2003 Jan;13(1):63–7.
4. Lopez Gil ML, Brimacombe J, Clar B. Sevoflurane versus propofol for induction and maintenance of anaesthesia with the laryngeal mask airway in children. *Paediatr Anaesth.* 1999;9(6):485–90.
5. Nakayama S, Furukawa H, Yanai H. Propofol reduces the incidence of emergence agitation in preschool-aged children as well as in school-aged children: a comparison with sevoflurane. *J Anesth.* 2007;21(1):19–23.
6. Kanaya A, Kuratani N, Satoh D, Kurosawa S. Lower incidence of emergence agitation in children after propofol anesthesia compared with sevoflurane: a meta-analysis of randomized controlled trials. *J Anesth.* 2014 Feb;28(1):4–11.
7. Vlajkovic GP, Sindjelic RP. Emergence delirium in children: many questions, few answers. *Anesth Analg.* 2007 Jan;104(1):84–91.
8. Bajwa SA, Costi D, Cyna AM. A comparison of emergence delirium scales following general anesthesia in children. *Paediatr Anaesth.* 2010 Aug;20(8):704–11.
9. Costi D, Cyna AM, Ahmed S, et al. Effects of sevoflurane versus other general anaesthesia on emergence agitation in children. *Cochrane Database Syst Rev.* 2014 Sep 12;9:CD007084.

INDEX